# NEW TRENDS IN NUCLEAR NEUROLOGY AND PSYCHIATRY

We pass and dream. Earth smiles. Virtue is rare.
Age, duty, gods weigh on our conscious bliss.
Hope for the best and for the worst prepare.
The sum of purposed wisdom speaks in this.

*Fernando Pessoa, Inscriptions in 'English Poems'*
*(b. 1888 - d. 1935)*

# NEW TRENDS IN NUCLEAR NEUROLOGY AND PSYCHIATRY

*Edited by*
*D.C. Costa*
*G.F. Morgan and*
*N.A. Lassen*

John Libbey

LONDON • PARIS • ROME

**British Library Cataloguing in Publication Data**

New Trends in Nuclear Neurology and Psychiatry
   I. Costa, D.C.
   616.89

ISBN: 0 86196 401 2

Published by

**John Libbey & Company Ltd,** 13 Smiths Yard, Summerley Street,
London SW18 4HR, England.
**Telephone: 081-947 2777 – Fax: 081-947 2664**
**John Libbey Eurotext Ltd,** 6 rue Blanche, 92120 Montrouge, France
**John Libbey - C.I.C. s.r.l.,** via Lazzaro Spallanzani 11, 00161 Rome, Italy

Printed in Great Britain by Ashford Colour Press Ltd,  Gosport, Hampshire,  UK.

# List of contributors

S. Asenbaum
Neurological University Clinic, Vienna, Austria

S. Aull
Neurological University Clinic, Vienna, Austria

Ch. Baumgartner
Neurological University Clinic, Vienna, Austria

Th. Brücke
Neurological University Clinic, Vienna, Austria

Durval Campos Costa
Institute of Nuclear Medicine, University College of London Medical School, London, UK

Michael D. Devous, Department of Radiology, University of Texas,
Southwestern Medical Center, Dallas, Texas, USA

Ferruccio Fazio
INB-CNR, Department of Nuclear Medicine, University of Milan,
Scientific Institute H. San Raffaele, Milan, Italy

Maria Carla Gilardi
INB-CNR, Department of Nuclear Medicine, University of Milan,
Scientific Institute H. San Raffaele, Milan, Italy

Peter H. Jarritt
Institute of Nuclear Medicine, University College of London Medical School, London, UK

Kypros Kouris
Institute of Nuclear Medicine, University College of London Medical School, London, UK

Niels A. Lassen
Dept. of Clinical Physiology/Nuclear Medicine, Bispebjerg Hospital,
DK-2400, Copenhagen N.V., Denmark

Giovanni Lucignani
INB-CNR, Department of Nuclear Medicine, University of Milan,
Scientific Institute H. San Raffaele, Milan, Italy

Bernard Mazière
Service Hospitalier Frédéric Joliot, Direction des Sciences du Vivant,
Commissariat à l'Energie Atomique, 91406 Orsay, France

Mariannick Mazière
Service Hospitalier Frédéric Joliot, Direction des Sciences du Vivant,
Commissariat à l'Energie Atomique, 91406 Orsay, France

Cristina Messa
INB-CNR, Department of Nuclear Medicine, University of Milan,
Scientific Institute H. San Raffaele, Milan, Italy

Rosa Maria Moresco
INB-CNR, Department of Nuclear Medicine, University of Milan,
Scientific Institute H. San Raffaele, Milan, Italy

Gill F. Morgan
Amersham International plc, Amersham Place, Little Chalfont,
Buckinghamshire, UK

Giovanni Paganelli
INB-CNR, Department of Nuclear Medicine, University of Milan,
Scientific Institute H. San Raffaele, Milan, Italy

Ivo Podreka
Neurological University Clinic, Vienna, Austria

Howard Ring
Lecturer in Neuropsychiatry, Institute of Neurology, Queen Square,
London WC1

Giovanna Rizzo
INB-CNR, Department of Nuclear Medicine, University of Milan,
Scientific Institute H. San Raffaele, Milan, Italy

Giuseppe Scotti
Department of Neuroradiology, University of Milan,
Scientific Institute H. San Raffaele, Milan, Italy

Fabio Triulzi
Department of Neuroradiology, University of Milan,
Scientific Institute H. San Raffaele, Milan, Italy

C. van der Meer
Neurological University Clinic, Vienna, Austria

Paul Verhoeff
Department of Nuclear Medicine, Academic Medical Centre,
Meibergdreef 9, 1105 AZ Amsterdam Zuidoost (NH), The Netherlands

S. Wenger
Neurological University Clinic, Vienna, Austria

# Contents

# Preface

There has been rapid recent growth in the number of radionuclide techniques used to aid the assessment of patients with neurological and psychiatric diseases. The investigation of regional brain perfusion and chemistry by means of tomographic techniques employing either single photon (SPET* or SPECT*) or positron (PET) emitters has led to a closer collaboration between neurologists and psychiatrists on the one hand and nuclear medicine physicians on the other. Furthermore, at every national or international scientific meeting on nuclear medicine techniques, a significant proportion of papers now deal with various aspects of the application of radionuclide methods to neurology and psychiatry.

The organizing committee of the 1992 annual congress of the European Association of Nuclear Medicine decided to give the title 'New Trends in Nuclear Neurology' to one of the post-congress meetings, held in Funchal, Madeira. The success of the lectures presented and the range of subjects covered, from the basic principles to the clinical applications of radionuclide methodology in neurology and psychiatry stimulated the production of the present volume. Instead of compiling the proceedings of the meeting we decided to produce a small book which will serve as a quick reference for those nuclear medicine physicians, particularly residents and young specialists, who decide to initiate their practice of nuclear neurology and psychiatry. At the same time we wanted to stimulate discussion of some issues of paramount importance for the present and future development of this interdisciplinary modality for the study of patients with diseases of the central nervous system.

By the time we had finished editing *New Trends in Nuclear Neurology and Psychiatry*, further research developments (regarding radiopharmaceuticals and instrumentation) and promising new clinical protocols had already emerged but could not be included. New ideas are constantly flowing from the creative imagination of those (scientists, clinical personnel and industry) striving to improve patient care, and particularly the diagnosis and therapeutic follow-up of neurological and psychiatric diseases. This opens the way for an editorial suggestion of continuation of this work beyond the 'decade of the brain' which would be reassuring for the future of nuclear medicine. Perhaps the EANM Committee on Nuclear Neurology and the organizing committees of future congresses will accept the challenge.

**D.C. Costa, G.F. Morgan and N. A. Lassen**

* Due to the non-uniformity of nomenclature, we decided to keep these two conventional designations as interchangeable until the nuclear medicine community accepts a single denomination.

# Foreword

SPECT functional brain imaging is a rapidly burgeoning field. As a satellite to the 1992 meeting of the European Association of Nuclear Medicine, leaders and learners in this exciting area met to share their views, concerns and expectations. The participants (hailing from throughout Europe and the United States) reflected the growing transatlantic collaboration that is essential to the future of nuclear medicine. Another collaboration important to our future was woven into the fabric of this post-congress meeting – the interaction between academia, industry and clinical practice. We are rapidly learning that our future lies in a partnership that crosses nations and oceans and that includes both the nuclear medicine community and our collaborating referrants in neurology and psychiatry.

The meeting was hosted by Durval C. Costa of the UCL Medical School, London. He, Gillian F. Morgan of Amersham International and Niels A. Lassen of Bispebjerg Hospital, Copenhagen serve as both editors of this book and as contributors. They have arranged herein overviews of fundamental principles (physiology, receptors, instrumentation and radiopharmaceuticals) and of clinical implementations.

The history of the measurement of regional cerebral blood flow (rCBF) with radio-isotopes is provided by Niels Lassen. The development of this technique from unidimensional to fully three-dimensional imaging modalities provides the reader with an excellent perspective of the rapid rate of growth that our field has experienced.

Durval Costa introduced the meeting and supplies in this volume his overview of the physiological basis underlying SPECT functional brain imaging. A thorough understanding of this basis is essential to proper use of the technique and interpretation of the resulting images. Both his perspective and carefully selected references should serve the reader well as foundational material.

Paul Verhoeff next reviews the fundamental bases of neuroreceptors. As such agents become increasingly available, it is important for us to understand receptor pharmacology and the basic principles underlying quantitation of receptor binding and kinetics. Several options for quantification of receptor density and receptor binding affinities are presented, with the advantages and disadvantages of each model well defined.

Peter Jarritt and Kypros Kouris provide a comprehensive review of the current state of SPECT instrumentation and compare the performance characteristics of a number of commercially available systems. Issues affecting image acquisition and processing, including display and quantification, are discussed and recommendations are offered for optimization of brain SPECT imaging procedures. Ours is a very dynamic field and this timely review of the state-of-the-art technology should be a valuable resource.

Gill Morgan and Durval Costa discuss the traditional blood–brain barrier radiopharmaceuticals (such as $^{99m}$Tc-DTPA and $^{99m}$Tc-glucoheptanoate in addition to radiopharmaceuticals used for the measurement of rCBF. It is fortunate that rCBF is so tightly coupled to cerebral metabolism in almost all circumstances and thus serves as a good marker of neuronal dysfunction. Also in this chapter the application of $^{201}$Tl to brain tumour imaging is reviewed. The growing diversity of available agents is an asset to the workers in this field and technical aspects of their design, pharmacokinetics and function are dealt with in this chapter.

Bernard and Mariannick Mazière address the challenge of describing the current and future clinical applications of SPECT receptor imaging. Many believe that much of our future rests in receptor imaging, which can likely be performed as effectively with SPECT as with PET but in a far more practical and affordable way. The authors' views clarify our current limitations (which are not so narrow as one might have thought) and highlight the areas of likely near term development.

The perspective of the neurological community is provided by Ivo Podreka and his collaborators. The use of SPECT in stroke, dementia and epilepsy are thoughtfully reviewed in his chapter. Clearly, these are the areas of greatest immediate clinical application and his considerable experience of brain SPECT imaging in the clinical setting lends authority to his recommendations.

The role of SPECT functional brain imaging in psychiatry is detailed by Howard Ring. He places a special emphasis on the role of activation studies which I believe will dominate the use of SPECT in psychiatry. Howard's observations hit the mark and clarify the future development of relevant clinical applications.

Finally, Giovanni Lucignani, heading the group from Milan, brings us back to our roots. Functional brain imaging often cannot be effectively interpreted in isolation. The role of structural brain imaging techniques, particularly magnetic resonance imaging (MRI), in detailing concurrent structural abnormalities is critical. He provides an excellent overview of the contribution from structural imaging to the diagnosis of those neurological and psychiatric disorders in which SPECT and PET play their most important roles. PET and SPECT are frequently complementary modalities which Giovanni compares in detail. He also provides insight into evolving MRI techniques for measuring brain function and the potential role for magnetic resonance spectroscopy (MRS).

The appendix comprises a number of characteristic images displaying brain perfusion patterns in normals and some classical pathological disease states.

It was our pleasure to share insights, meet new friends and re-establish old connections in Funchal, the capital city of the beautiful Portuguese island of Madeira. In a setting rich with history and overgrown with nature's beauty, both our spirit and our intellect were nourished under the equatorial sun. While the reader of this volume will miss Madeira's charm, we hope that the intellectual environment provided will be as stimulating as the original. Certainly, both the editors and the authors are to be congratulated for their fine effort. ·

**Michael D. Devous, Sr., Ph.D.**
**Associate Professor of Radiology, University of Texas**
**Southwestern Medical Center**
**Dallas, Texas, USA**

# *Section I*
# HISTORICAL BACKGROUND

The most important historical landmarks leading to the development and application of radionuclide methods in the evaluation of patients with neuropsychiatric diseases are described.

Several radiopharmaceuticals have been utilized to assess cerebral functions in man. Two of them, $^{133}$Xe and $^{99m}$Tc-HMPAO, enabled the use of widespread routine clinical protocols to investigate regional cerebral blood flow (rCBF).

In this section, Niels A. Lassen describes the historical sequence of events that originated rCBF mapping with $^{133}$Xe[2,3] and with $^{99m}$Tc-HMPAO after the first report of its use in man by Ell *et al.* in 1985[1].

1. Ell, P.J., Cullum, I., Costa, D.C., Jarritt, P.H., Hocknell, J.M.L., Lui, D., Jewkes, R.F., Steiner, T.J., Nowotnik, D.P., Pickett, R.D. & Neirinckx, R.D. (1985): A new regional Cerebral Blood flow Mapping with Tc-99m-labelled Compound. *Lancet* **ii,** 50–51.

2. Lassen, N.A., Ingvar, D.H. & Skinhøj, E. (1978): Brain function and blood flow. Changes in the amount of blood flowing in areas of the human cortex, reflecting changes in the activity of those areas, are graphically revealed with the aid of radioactive isotopes. *Sci. Am.* **239,** 62–71.

3. Mallett, B.L. & Veall, N. (1963): Investigation of cerebral blood flow in hypertension, using radioactive Xenon inhalation and extracranial recording. *Lancet* **i,** 1081–1082.

*New Trends in Nuclear Neurology and Psychiatry*, edited by D.C. Costa, G.F. Morgan and N. A. Lassen
© 1993 John Libbey & Company Ltd., pp. 3–13

# Chapter 1

# On the history of measurement of cerebral blood flow in man by radioactive isotopes

Niels A. Lassen

*Dept. of Clinical Physiology/Nuclear Medicine, Bispebjerg Hospital, DK-2400 Copenhagen N.V., Denmark*

Lassen and Munck started in 1952 in Copenhagen to use $^{85}$Kr instead of nitrous oxide for measuring CBF by the Kety–Schmidt technique. We reported our preliminary experience at the Seventh International Congress of Radiology held in Copenhagen 19–25 July 1953[33], but a full report appeared first in 1955[34]. Also in 1955, Landau, Freygang, Rowland, Sokoloff and Kety published their autoradiographic method for measuring regional CBNF in animals using $^{131}$I-trifluoro-methane[28], an approach that was applied later for measuring regional CBF in man by PET or SPECT. Even with respect to non-diffusible tracers 1955 is noteworthy, as this year Nylin & Blömer first used a radioactive tracer for measuring CBF in man by the dye dilution principle[40,41].

Thus, practically speaking, we may set 1955 as the year when the use of radioactive isotopes for measuring CBF started. Radioactive isotopes have since played a dominant role for the development of clinically useful CBF methods based on SPECT or PET. This paper will outline this development. The chronological approach is not chosen, as the material is arranged according to the basic methodological principle involved.

## One-dimensional CBF (global values)

In 1944 Seymour S. Kety, working in Carl F. Schmidt's laboratory in Philadelphia, developed the nitrous oxide method for measuring CBF in man. His method is based on inhalation of an inert gas and on collecting multiple samples of arterial blood and of venous blood draining the brain (Fig. 1). The method was published in 1945 by Kety & Schmidt in their classic paper and it was the first allowing accurate physiological and clinical studies of flow and metabolism in the brain[23]. Kety & Schmidt co-authored the first several papers and it became known therefore as the Kety–Schmidt technique. Schmidt has given a brief account of the early years acknowledging Kety's essential role in proposing and implementing the basic principle[53]. The technique allows simultaneous measurement of the arteriovenous differences for oxygen and glucose, and by multiplying CBF by (A-V)$_{O2}$ or (A-V)$_{glu}$ the metabolic rates for oxygen or glucose are obtained.

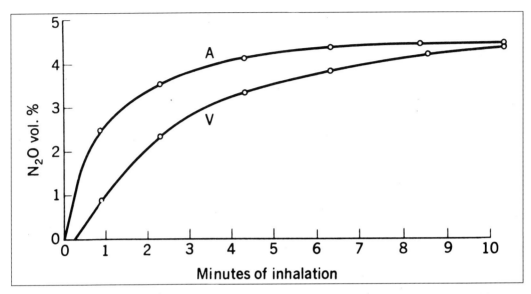

Fig. 1. Determination of global cerebral blood flow in man with nitrous oxide. Curves obtained by Kety in first study on July 1944, in patient with hypertension. CBF is 57.5 ml/100 g/min. (From Fishman, A.P. & Richards, D.W., Circulation of the Blood, Men and Ideas, Oxford, Oxford University Press, 1965).

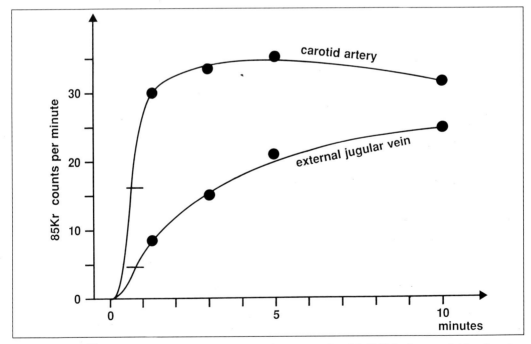

Fig. 2. First [85]Kr saturation curves obtained in a dog on October 24, 1952 by Lassen & Munck and used in grant application to develop a practical counting system to be used for the routine studies in man reported at an international congress in July, 1953[33] and published as a scientific paper in 1955[34].

Kety & Schmidt used nitrous oxide as the inert gas and studied the saturation of the brain for 10 min. Radioactive inert gases however afford the advantage of increasing accuracy of measurement. They were first introduced in 1955 by Lassen & Munck using $^{85}$Kr[34] (see Fig. 2). However, the analytical procedure was simplified using $^{133}$Xe as described by Astrup *et al.* [1] These authors administered xenon gas by continuous intravenous infusion and studied CBF during the desaturation phase. This modification combined with correction for the lack of complete equilibrium probably constitutes the most accurate approach existing, the 'gold standard' of global CBF measurement[36]. It yields average values of $46 \pm 9$ ml/100 g/min for CBF, of $3.0 \pm 0.4$ ml/100 g/min for CMRO$_2$, and of $24 \pm 3$ mol/100 g/min for CMR$_{Gluc}$ in young, normal adults. A less accurate but completely atraumatic approach for measuring global CBF is to use the average value of the regional CBFs obtained using $^{133}$Xe inhalation and stationary detectors. This method, discussed in the next section, is particularly suited for serial CBF studies that cannot readily be implemented by the Kety–Schmidt method.

**Two-dimensional CBF (side views)**

Inhalation of $^{133}$Xe combined with a battery of stationary scintillation detectors has been used extensively to study regional CBF, since the pioneer studies of Mallett & Veall[37]. Usually the detectors are placed laterally over the side of the head, but a radial arrangement has also been employed. The most advanced instrumentation, consisting of 254 small detectors, was developed by Risberg[51] in 1987.

Methodological improvements of the $^{133}$Xe-inhalation-external-counting method have been introduced in particular by Risberg *et al.*, who in 1975 described the so-called 'initial slope index' as a reliable parameter, that closely relates to the mean value for CBF[52]. The many contributions by Obrist and co-workers starting in 1967 have also been of major importance (cf. Obrist & Wilkinson[44]). It should be stressed, however, that the method suffers from unavoidable errors involved in assessing the input function[43] and errors due to $^{133}$Xe uptake in the nasal sinuses and in the soft tissues outside the brain[38]. These so-called 'extra-cerebral contaminations' and the very limited resolution in depth mean that regional information of CBF is blurred to a considerable extent, invalidating the method for the study of localized brain diseases such as stroke or focal epilepsy. Patients with severe lung disease cannot be reliably studied either. Despite these shortcomings the $^{133}$Xe-inhalation-external-counting method can be considered to be the method of choice in certain contexts. As already mentioned, the method is probably the best for studying CBF changes in normal man over many days using average changes in 'initial slope index' of all detectors to indicate changes in CBF. The amount of $^{133}$Xe can be kept so low that five or even 10 studies can be carried out per person without the radiation exposure exceeding the level considered acceptable in normal adults.

Two-dimensional CBF data with better spatial resolution are obtained when administering the radioactive inert gas intra-arterially as a bolus of the gas dissolved in saline, an approach first described by Lassen & Ingvar in 1961 using $^{85}$Kr[20,31].

The inert gas most widely used with this method is $^{133}$Xe introduced by Harper *et al.* in 1964[13]. $^{15}$O-labelled H$_2$O has only been used by a single group[9]. Also confined to a single group was the ingenious use of $^{81m}$Kr infusion, a technique giving a steady-state image that almost matches rCBF distribution because of the short half-life of the isotope[11]. The intra-arterial inert gas injection method was analysed in detail by Høedt-Rasmussen and co-workers in 1966[18] and by Olesen *et al.* in 1971[48]. In the latter paper the authors propose the initial slope as a reliable and easily measured index of the blood flow in the cerebral cortex. Using this approach Olesen in 1971 published, from this author's laboratory, the first definite evidence of focal CBF increase

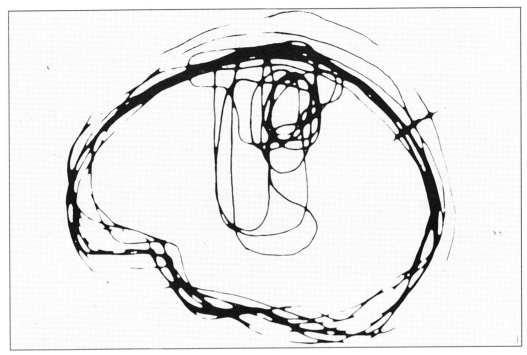

*Fig. 3. Area of contralateral cortical flow increase ('focal' activation of CBF) seen with unilateral hand movement[47].*

in the human brain elicited by neuronal activity: a contralateral focal increase of regional CBF was observed when working with one hand[47] (see Fig. 3).

'The first observation was made fortuitously. We intended to increase the blood pressure in a subject in order to study autoregulation of CBF. As we did not want to use drugs for raising the pressure, we had the subject performing ischaemic exercise. This involved the blowing up of an arm cuff to suprasystolic pressure levels and having the subject open and clench his fist rhythmically to the point of pain and ischaemic paralysis. It was our good luck, that we had him use the hand opposite the detector system. Comparing the $^{133}$Xe washout curves to those obtained at rest 15 min before, we noted to our great surprise a CBF increase of about 50 per cent in the upper central part of the hemisphere – in the primary sensory motor hand area controlling the opposite hand's movements.

'In a way, we should not have been so surprised. Sokoloff had already in 1961 reported marked flow increases in the visual cortex of cats during photic stimulation[54]. Yet, we *were* surprised – having by then already worked with the intra-arterial method for measuring cortex CBF in man for 10 years, without ever suspecting that the functional activity of the cortex mattered, and then suddenly being made aware of our mistake in a most convincing way.'

Mapping active brain areas by CBF during various sensory and motor stimulation was subsequently undertaken by our group in collaboration with D.H. Ingvar in Lund, Sweden. Of particular importance for these studies was the computer-based 256 detector system for measuring CBF developed in 1973 by Sveinsdottir & Lassen[58], the system which introduced the now so familiar colour coding of the numerical data to facilitate the visual analysis. A review of these findings published in 1978 in *Scientific American* by Lassen, Ingvar & Skinhøj opened up the field of studying local brain activity by mapping CBF[32].

This approach has since then been assiduously studied in particular by positron tomography. The intra-carotid [133]Xe injection method is today no longer used clinically because of the potential hazard it involves. It should be emphasized, however, that much of the basic knowledge about CBF in disease states was obtained through this method during the 20 years it was in use. An early result was the description of reflow hyperaemia in ischaemic infarcts due to spontaneous thrombolysis published by Lassen in 1966, who dubbed it 'luxury perfusion' to stress that flow was greatly in excess of the metabolic need of the evolving infarct[29]. The frequent occurrence of this type of hyperaemia was documented by several groups[7,12,19].

Non-diffusible radioactive tracers have been used in many studies to follow the passage of the blood through the brain, an approach introduced by Eichhorn in 1957[8], by Oldendorf *et al.* in 1960[46], and by Fazio & Fieschi in 1960[10]. Using a gamma camera, a crude cerebral angiogram is obtained. The approach has, however, contributed little clinically or theoretically to the study of CBF. Many attempts have been made to quantitate the transit of such tracers in terms of CBF, but no reliable method has resulted. This topic will, therefore, not be discussed further.

**Three-dimensional CBF (tomography)**

Tomographic reconstruction of radioisotope distribution was described as a principle in 1961 by Oldendorf[45]. Subsequently emission tomography was developed into a clinical tool by Kuhl and Edwards in a series of papers of which the first was published in 1963[25,26,27]. Kuhl and Edwards used conventional gamma emitting isotopes and are thus the fathers of SPECT. The same principle was applied to positron scintigraphy in 1971 by Chesler[3]. The development of emission tomography thus antedates, by many years, the epoch making and completely independent application of the same principles to X-ray transmission tomography ('CT-scanning') by Hounsfield[17] and Cormack[6] in 1973.

The first tomographic method for CBF measurement by SPECT was developed by Lassen *et al.* in 1978 using [133]Xe gas administered by inhalation[35,57]. The method is completely atraumatic, as it essentially is a tomographic version of the two-dimensional [133]Xe inhalation approach. Due to the rapidly changing concentration of the tracer in the brain this approach necessitated the development of a highly sensitive and rapidly rotating SPECT instrument of the type Tomomatic[35,57] or Headtome[59]. Recently Coppola *et al.* used [127]Xe as the inert gas[5]. This tracer allows improved spatial resolution without increasing the radiation exposure.

Tracers retained in the brain tissue in the pattern of CBF have been described more recently. Three classes of such tracers can be discerned: [123]I-labelled amines as developed by Winchell *et al.* (1980) with [123]I-iodo-isopropyl-amphetamine (IMP) being the most prominent member of this class[61,62]; [201]Tl-labelled diethyldithiocarbamate (DDC) developed by Bruine *et al.* in 1985[2]; [99m]Tc-labelled compounds as hexamethylpropyleneamineoxime (HMPAO) described by Nowotnik *et al.* in 1985[39] and ethyl-cysteinate-dimer (ECD) described by Walovitch in 1988[60].

A tracer which is retained by the brain allows imaging of CBF distribution to be performed by conventional rotating gamma camera systems. They have given an explosive impetus to the clinical use of CBF studies, a topic beyond the scope of this historically oriented review. It is appropriate to mention, however, that with all these tracers the retention in the brain depends on chemical properties of the brain tissue that may be altered (as for example in infarct tissue). With [99m]Tc-HMPAO (and also with [99m]Tc-ECD) the distribution image is not completely linear with respect to CBF, as incomplete extraction and early back-diffusion is most marked in high flow areas. A simple algorithm allowing to correct for this error was developed by Lassen *et al.* in

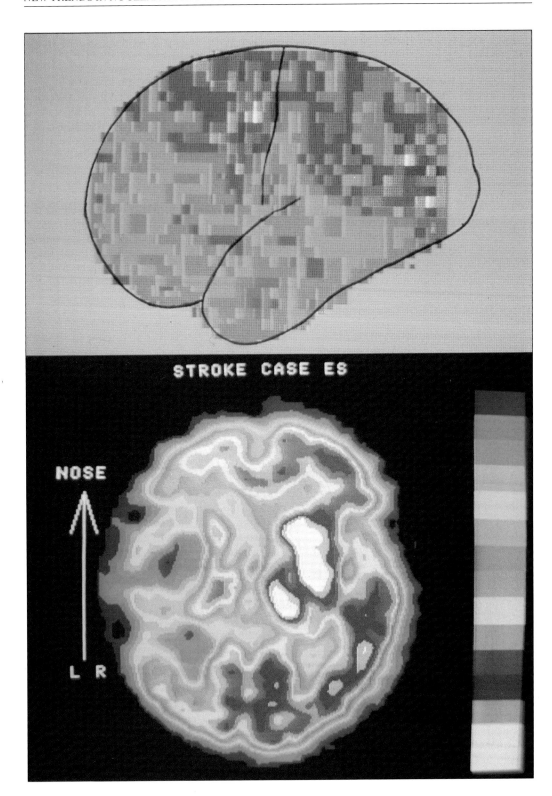

*Upper Illustration:*

$^{133}$*Xe intra-carotid injection CBF during visual perception of moving object – the finger of the investigator (Lassen, Ingvar, Skinhøj, in 1978). Each colour step corresponds to a 6% change in CBF relative to the resting state with closed, non-moving eyes, lightest blue colour denotes no change. Side view of normal left hemisphere, frontal lobe towards the left.*

*Flow increase of 18–30 per cent is seen in visual association cortex (towards the left) in the frontal eye field (in middle) and in supplementary motor area (slightly towards the right and at upper edge).*

*Lower Illustration:*

$^{99m}$*Tc-HMPAO by i.v. injection for measuring CBF by SPECT. Image shows 'slice' through basal ganglia with approx. 8 mm spatial resolution (FWHM) obtained in a patient with ischaemic stroke studied by the four-headed SPECT system developed in 1978 by Lassen et al.[35] by applying the principles pioneered by Kuhl & Edwards in 1963[25].*

*Commentary:*

*Kety & Schmidt used 15 per cent nitrous oxide as the inert gas. It has no discernible biological effects and 15 per cent $N_2O$ can consequently be considered as a tracer. But $N_2O$ analysis in blood samples involves extraction of the gas and is cumbersome and technically demanding. With radioactive inert gases the tracer concentration can be measured without extracting the gas from the blood. This increases the accuracy and the extrapolation to full saturation, as already proposed by Kety & Schmidt in 1945, and becomes sufficiently accurate to be implemented routinely as shown by Lassen & Munck in 1955. Extrapolation corrects for uneven flows in the brain, a factor which, according to Ogden & Sapirstein's classic paper from 1956 must be considered to be the theoretical main source of error – the Achilles heel – of the Kety–Schmidt technique. For these reasons the author is of the opinion, that the radioactive inert gas version of the Kety–Schmidt technique constitutes the 'gold standard' for global values. A more detailed discussion of these problems has recently been published by Madsen et al. (1993).*

*The desaturation approach results in very precise inert gas curves. Combining this with slow intravenous infusion of the gas dissolved in saline to attain near full saturation obviates the use of a face mask that constitutes on a practical level the biggest source of error of the Kety–Schmidt technique which arises due to leakage of air.*

1988[30]. For absolute quantitation it is probably best to scale the HMPAO image to the global CBF measured by [133]Xe inhalation (see above).

Tomographic measurements of CBF by PET were first described by Jones *et al.* in 1976[21] using infusion of [15]O-labelled water. A number of modifications of the method has been described and in particular bolus injection of [15]O-H$_2$O has become widely used since the approach was described in 1983 by the PET group in St. Louis[14,49]. Theoretically water is not an ideal tracer for CBF, as its unidirectional extraction across the blood–brain barrier is not 100 per cent. In particular at very high flow values a moderate degree of flow-limitation will occur[9]. For this reason other positron-labelled diffusible tracers have been developed for CBF measurement in man such as [77]Kr developed by Hondayer *et al.* in 1977[16] or [11]C-butanol implemented by Herscovitch *et al.* in 1987[15].

## Concluding comments

The sensitivity of detecting radioactivity permits us to study smaller concentrations of chemical substances than is available to us with other classical techniques of detection. This aspect is specifically explored in the methods developed for studying brain metabolism or neuroreceptors with radioisotopes. Tomographic measurement of regional CMRO$_2$ by PET was first described by Jones *et al.* in 1976 in the same paper in which they introduced their tomographic CBF method[21]. Also in 1976 Reivich published the principle of the [18]F-deoxyglucose method for measuring regional CMR$_{glucose}$ in man[50], a method developed on the basis of Sokoloff's [14]C-deoxyglucose method for animal studies developed in 1974[22,55,56].

Neuroreceptor studies based on positron-emitting tracers have evolved rapidly since Kook *et al.* in 1975[24] described the synthesis of [18]F-haloperidol, which is mainly a dopamine type-D$_2$ ligand. Particular success has been obtained with ligands binding to the central benzodiazepine receptor, a development that started in 1979 when Comar *et al.* synthesized [11]C-flunitrazepam[4]. Several hundreds of labelled ligands for PET or SPECT must by now have been produced and the biological behaviour of many of them has been studied in detail. Yet, their clinical usefulness is still unclear and largely unexplored. Therefore, over the next few years to come more clinically oriented neuroreceptor studies will probably appear. Meanwhile routine CBF studies by SPECT is increasingly used in larger hospital ·centres, as their practical value is becoming widely recognized – in particular in some stroke cases, in milder forms of Alzheimer's diseases and other types of dementia, and in focal epilepsy.

## References

1. Astrup, J., Rosenørn, J., Cold, G.E., Bendtsen, A. & Sorensen, P.M. (1984): Minimum cerebral blood flow and metabolism during craniotomy. Effect of thiopental loading. *Acta Anaesthesiol. Scand.* **28**, 478–481.

2. Bruine, J., van Royen, E., Vyth, A., deJong, J.M.B.V. & van der Schoot, J.B. (1985): Thallium-201 diethyldithio-carbamate: an alternative to iodine-123 *n*-isopropyl-*p*-iodoamphetamine. *J. Nucl. Med.* **26**, 925–929.

3. Chesler, D.A. (1973): Positron tomography and three dimensional reconstruction techniques. In: *Tomographic imaging in nuclear medicine*, ed. G.S. Freedman, pp. 176–183. New York: Society of Nuclear Medicine.

4. Comar, D., Zarifian, E., Verhas, M., Soussaline, F., Mazière, M., Berger, G., Loo, H., Cuche, H., Kellershohn, C. & Deniker, P. (1979): Brain distribution and kinetics of [11]C-chlorpromazine in schizophrenics: positron emission tomography studies. *Psychiatry Res.* **1**, 23–29.

5. Coppola, R., Marenco, S., Jones, D.W., David D.G. & Weinberger, D.R. (1990): Assessment of [133]Xe as a dynamic SPECT rCBF tracer in normal subjects at rest. *Soc. Neurosci. Abs.* **16**, 23.

6. Cormack, A.M. (1973): Reconstruction of densities from their projections, with applications in radiological physics. *Phys. Med. Biol.* **18**, 195–207.

7.  Cronqvist, S. & Laroche, F. (1967): Transitory 'hyperemia' in focal cerebral vascular lesions studied by angiography and regional cerebral blood flow measurements. *Brit. J. Rad. Diagn.* **7**, 521–525.

8.  Eichhorn, O. (1957): Zur Objektivierung zerebraler Durchblutungsschäden im höheren Lebensalter. *Verh. Dtsch Ges. Kreislaufforsch* **24**, 253–258.

9.  Eichling, J.O., Raichle, M.E., Grubb Jr, R.I. & Ter-Pogossian, M.M. (1974): Evidence of the limitations of water as a freely diffuseable tracer in brain of the rhesus monkey. *Circ. Res.* **35**, 358–364.

10. Fazio, C. & Fieschi, C. (1960): Valutazione dell'emodinamica cerebrale con isotopi radioattivi. *Minerva Nucleare* **4**, 323–341.

11. Fazio, F., Fieschi, C., Nardini, M. & Forli, C. (1977): Assessment of rCBF by continuous infusion of $^{81m}$Kr. *J. Nucl. Med.* **18**, 962–966.

12. Fieschi, C., Agnoli, A., Battistini, N. & Bozzao, L. (1966): Regional cerebral blood flow in patients with brain infarcts. *Arch. Neurol.* **15**, 653–663.

13. Harper, A.M., Glass, H.I., Steven, J.L. & Granat, A.H. (1964): The measurement of local blood flow in the cerebral cortex from the clearance of Xenon-133. *J. Neurol. Neurosurg. Psychiatry* **27**, 255–258.

14. Herscovitch, P., Markham, J. & Raichle, M.E. (1983): Brain blood flow measured with intravenous H$_2$ $^{15}$O. I. Theory and error analysis. *Nucl. Med.* **24**, 782–789.

15. Herscovitch, P., Raichle, M., Kilbourn, M.R. & Welch, M.J. (1987): Positron emission tomography measurements of cerebral blood flow and permeability-surface area product of water using $^{15}$O-water and $^{11}$C-butanol. *J. Cereb. Blood Flow Metab.* **7**, 527–542.

16. Hondayer, A.J., Meyer, E. & Yamamoto, Y.L. (1977): Cyclotron production of Krypton-77 for regional cerebral blood flow measurement. *Int. J. Nucl. Med. Biol.* **4**, 83–85.

17. Hounsfield, G.N. (1973): Computerized transverse axial scanning (tomography): Part 1: Description of system. *Br. J. Radiol.* **46**, 1016–1020.

18. Høedt-Rasmussen, K., Sveinsdottir, E. & Lassen, N.A. (1966): Regional cerebral blood flow in man determined by intra-arterial injection of radioactive inert gas. *Circ. Res.* **18**, 237–247.

19. Høedt-Rasmussen, K., Skinhøj, E., Paulson, O., Ewald, J., Bjerrum, K., Fahrenkrug, A. & Lassen, N.A. (1967): Regional cerebral blood flow in acute apoplexy. The 'luxury perfusion syndrome' of brain tissue. *Arch. Neurol.* **17**, 271–281.

20. Ingvar, D.H. & Lassen, N.A. (1961): Quantitative determination of regional cerebral blood flow in man. *Lancet* **ii**, 806–807.

21. Jones, T., Chesler, D.A. & Ter-Pogossian, M.M. (1976): The continuous inhalation of oxygen is for assessing regional oxygen extraction in the brain of man. *Br. J. Radiol.* **49**, 339–343.

22. Kennedy, C., Des Rosiers, M.H., Jehle, J.W., Reivich, M., Sharpe, F. & Sokoloff, L. (1975): Mapping of functional neural pathways by autoradiographic survey of local metabolic rate with [$^{14}$C]deoxyglucose. *Science* **187**, 850–853.

23. Kety, S.S. & Schmidt, C.F. (1945): The determination of cerebral blood flow in man by the use of nitrous oxide in low concentrations. *Am. J. Physiol.* **143**, 53–66.

24. Kook, C.S., Reed, M.F. & Digenis, G.A. (1975): Preparation of [$^{18}$F]haloperidol. *J. Med. Chem.* **18**, 533–535.

25. Kuhl, D.E. & Edwards, R.Q. (1963): Image separation radioisotope scanning. *Radiology* **80**, 653–662.

26. Kuhl, D.E. & Edwards, R.Q. (1970): The Mark III scanner. A compact device for multiple-view and section scanning of the brain. *Radiology* **96**, 563–570.

27. Kuhl, D.E., Edwards, R.Q., Ricci, A.R. & Reivich, M. (1973): Quantitative section scanning using orthogonal tangent correction. *J. Nucl. Med.* **14**, 196–200.

28. Landau, W.M., Freygang, W.H. Jr, Rowland, L.P., Sokoloff, L. & Kety, S.S. (1955): The local circulation of the living brain: values in the unanesthetised and anesthetised cat. *Trans. Am. Neurol. Assoc.* **80**, 125–129.

29. Lassen, N.A. (1966): The luxury perfusion syndrome and its possible relation to acute metabolic acidosis localised within the brain. *Lancet* **ii**, 1113–1115.

30. Lassen, N.A., Andersen, A.R., Friberg, L. & Paulson, O.B. (1988): The retention of [$^{99m}$Tc]-d,l-HMPAO in the human brain after intracarotid bolus injection: kinetic analysis. *J. Cereb. Blood Flow Metab.* **8**, S13–S22.

31. Lassen, N.A. & Ingvar, D.H. (1961): The blood flow of the cerebral cortex determined by radioactive Krypton-85. *Experientia* **17**, 42–45.

32.    Lassen, N.A., Ingvar, D.H. & Skinhøj, E. (1978): Brain function and blood flow. Changes in the amount of blood flowing in areas of the human cerebral cortex, reflecting changes in the activity of those areas, are graphically revealed with the aid of radioactive isotopes. *Sci. Am.* **239**, 62–71.

33.    Lassen, N.A. & Munck, O. (1953): The cerebral blood flow in man determined by the use of radioactive Krypton-85. Paper presented at the Seventh International Congress of Radiology, Copenhagen, Denmark, 19–24 July, 1953.

34.    Lassen, N.A. & Munck, O. (1955): The cerebral blood flow in man determined by the use of radioactive Krypton. *Acta Physiol. Scand.* **33**, 30–49.

35.    Lassen, N.A., Sveinsdottir, E., Kanno, I., Stokely, E.M. & Rommer P. (1978): A fast moving, single photon emission tomograph for regional cerebral blood flow studies in man (Abstr.) *J. Comput. Assist. Tomogr.* **2**, 661–662.

36.    Madsen, P.L., Holm, S., Herning, M., & Lassen, N.A. (1993): Average blood flow and oxygen uptake in the human brain during resting wakefulness, A critical praisal of the Kety–Schmidt technique. *J. Cereb. Blood Flow Metab.* (in press).

37.    Mallett, B.L. & Veall, N. (1963): Investigation of cerebral blood-flow in hypertension, using radioactive-Xenon inhalation and extracranial recording. *Lancet* **i**, 1081–1082.

38.    Nilsson, B.G., Ryding, E. & Ingvar, D.H. (1982): Quantitative airway artefact compensation at regional cerebral blood flow measurements with radioactive gases. *J. Cereb. Blood Flow Metab.* **2**, 73–78.

39.    Nowotnik, D.P., Canning, L.R., Cumming, S.A., Harrison, R.C., Higley, B., Nechvatal, G. Pickett R.D., Piper, I.M., Bayne, V.J., Forster, A.M., Weisner, P.S. & Neirinckx, R.D. (1985): Development of a $^{99m}$Tc-labelled radiopharmaceutical for cerebral blood flow imaging. *Nucl. Med. Commun.* **6**, 499–506.

40.    Nylin, G. & Blömer, H. (1955): Studien über die zerebrale zirculation mit radioactiven Isotopen. *Zschr. Kreislaufforsch* **44**, 139–143.

41.    Nylin, G. & Blömer, H. (1955): Studies on distribution of cerebral blood flow with thorium B-labelled erythrocytes. *Circ. Res.* **3**, 79–8

42.    Obrist, W.D., Thompson, H.K., King, C.H. & Wang, H.S. (1967): Determinations of regional cerebral blood flow by inhalation of Xenon-133. *Circ. Res.* **20**, 124–135.

43.    Obrist, W.D., Wilkinson, W.E., Wang, H.S. & Harel, D. (1988): The noninvasive $^{133}$Xe method: influence of the input function on computed rCBF values. In: *Handbook of regional cerebral blood flow*, eds. S. Knezevic, V.A. Maximilian, S. Mubrin, I. Prohovnik & J. Wade, pp. 37–50: Lawrence Erlbaum.

44.    Obrist, W.D. & Wilkinson, W.E. (1990): Regional cerebral blood flow measurement in humans by Xenon-133 clearance. *Brain Metab. Rev.* **2**, 283–327.

45.    Oldendorf, W.H. (1961): Isolated flying spot detection of radiodensity discontinuities – displaying the internal structural patterns of a complex object. *IRE Trans. Bio-Med. Elect. BME* **8**, 68–72.

46.    Oldendorf, W.H., Crandall, P.H., Nordyke, R.A. & Rose, A.S. (1960): A comparison of the arrival in the cerebral hemispheres of intravenously injected radioisotope. *Neurology* **10**, 223–227.

47.    Olesen, J. (1971): Contralateral focal increase of cerebral blood flow in man during arm work. *Brain* **94**, 635–646.

48.    Olesen, J., Paulson, O.B. & Lassen, N.A. (1971): Regional cerebral blood flow in man determined by the initial slope of the clearance of intra-arterially injected $^{133}$Xe. *Stroke* **2**, 519–540.

49.    Raichle, M.E., Martin, W.R.W., Herscovitch, P., Mintun, M.A. & Markham, J. (1983): Brain blood flow measured with intravenous $H_2$ $^{15}$O. II. Implementation and validation. *J. Nucl. Med.* **24**, 790–798.

50.    Reivich, M. (1976): Application of the deoxyglucose method to human cerebral dysfunction. The use of [2-$^{18}$F]Fluoro-2-deoxy-D-glucose in man: *Neurosci Res. Program Bull.,* **14**, 502–504.

51.    Risberg, J. (1987): Development of high-resolution two-dimensional measurement of regional cerebral blood flow. In: *Impact of functional imaging in neurology and psychiatry*, eds. J. Wade, S. Knezevic, V.A. Maximilian, Z. Mubrin & I. Prohovnik, pp. 35–43. London: John Libbey.

52.    Risberg, J., Ali, Z., Wilson, E.M., Wills, E.L. & Halsey, J.H. (1975): Regional cerebral blood flow by $^{133}$Xenon inhalation: preliminary evaluation of an initial slope index in patients with unstable flow compartments. *Stroke* **6**, 142–148.

53.    Schmidt, C.F. (1982): The early days of the indifferent gas method for measuring cerebral blood flow. *J. Cereb. Blood Flow Metab.* **2**, 1–2.

54.   Sokoloff, L. (1961): Local cerebral circulation at rest and during altered cerebral activity induced by anesthesia or visual stimulation. In: *Regional neurochemistry*, eds. S.S. Kety & J. Elkes. Oxford: Pergamon Press.

55.   Sokoloff, L., Reivich, M., Patlak, C.S., Petticrew, K.D., Des Rosiers, M. & Kennedy, C. (1974): The [$^{14}$C]deoxyglucose method for the quantitative determination of local cerebral glucose consumption. *Trans. Am. Soc. Neurochem.* **5**, 85 (abstr).

56.   Sokoloff, L., Reivich, M., Kennedy, C., Des Rosiers, M.H., Patlak, C.S., Pettigrew, K.D. Sakurada, O. & Shinohara, M. (1977): The [$^{14}$C]deoxyglucose method for the measurement of local cerebral glucose utilization: theory, procedure, and normal values in the conscious and anesthetized albino rat. *J. Neurochem.* **28**, 897–916.

57.   Stokely, E.M., Sveinsdottir, E., Lassen, N.A. & Rommer, P. (1980): A single photon dynamic computer-assisted tomograph (DCAT) for imaging brain function in multiple cross-sections. *J. Comput. Assist. Tomogr.* **4**, 230–240.

58.   Sveinsdottir, E. & Lassen, N.A. (1975): A 254-detector system for measuring regional cerebral blood flow. In: *Cerebral circulation & metabolism*, eds. T.W. Langfitt, L.C. McHenry Jr, M. Reivich & H. Wollman), pp. 414–418. Berlin: Springer.

59.   Tanaka, M., Hirose, Y., Koga, K. & Hattori, H. (1981): Engineering aspects of a hybrid emission computed tomograph. *IEEE Trans. Nucl. Sci.* NS-28, 137–141.

60.   Walovitch, R.C., Hall, K.M., O'Toole, J.J. & Williams, S.J. (1988): Metabolism of $^{99m}$Tc-ECD in normal volunteers. *J. Nucl. Med.* **29**, Abstr. 27, p. 747.

61.   Winchell, H.S., Baldwin, R.M. & Lin, T.H. (1980): Development of $^{123}$I-labelled amines for brain studies: localization of $^{123}$I-iodophenylalkyl amines in rat brain. *J. Nucl. Med.* **21**, 940–946.

62.   Winchell, H.S., Horst, W.D., Braun, L., Oldendorf, N.H., Hattner, W.H. & Parker, H. (1980): N-Isopropyl-[$^{123}$I]-p-iodoamphetamine: single-pass brain uptake and washout; binding to brain synaptosomes; and localization in dog and monkey brain. *J. Nucl. Med.* **21**, 947–952.

# Section II
# PHYSIOLOGICAL BASIS FOR BRAIN IMAGING WITH RADIONUCLIDES

The complex organization of the central nervous system has for decades challenged scientists and their ability to understand first the gross and microscopic anatomy and more recently neurophysiology and disease processes.

In the practice of neurology, the physical signs discovered during patient examination usually indicate with great precision the anatomical localization of the lesion or lesions responsible for the functional abnormalities present. A detailed history of the disease often discloses the sequence and evolution of the symptoms and thus gives an indication of the nature of the pathological process. In situations like this, nuclear medicine with its radionuclide methodology, mainly functional, has little to offer. However, there are neurological disorders with a clear and typical clinical picture (if patients are good observers) and very poor or completely negative physical examination. Migraine, epilepsy and some degenerative diseases are characteristic examples. In these conditions with little or no structural abnormality easily identifiable, the radionuclide methodology has recently been playing an important role either using positron (PET) or single photon emitters (SPET). Moreover, psychiatrists all over the world are becoming more than ever interested in the so-called 'biological psychiatry'. They try to understand behavioural and mood changes in their patients better than previously. There are many theories based on neurotransmitters that seem to be able to explain certain aspects of psychiatric diseases better than pure psychological theories.

Brain perfusion studies and investigation of the availability of neuroreceptors are now important tools for research and clinical studies in neurology and psychiatry.

This section deals with the basic knowledge from the vascular supply to the brain fixation of radiotracers for brain imaging with a special reference to the barriers from blood to meninges and brain, as well as the biochemical processes behind neurotransmission.

*New Trends in Nuclear Neurology and Psychiatry*, edited by D.C. Costa, G.F. Morgan and N. A. Lassen
© 1993 John Libbey & Company Ltd., pp. 17–24

# Chapter 2

# Cerebral blood flow, blood–brain barrier

Durval Campos Costa

*Institute of Nuclear Medicine, University College of London Medical School, London, UK*

## Introduction

In order to be able to contribute to a better evaluation of the neuropsychiatric patient, nuclear medicine physicians need to have a good knowledge of the basic neuroanatomy and physiology, in addition to the pharmacokinetic and pharmacodynamic factors affecting the distribution, uptake/retention and utilization of radiotracers by the nervous system in general and the brain in particular.

In general pharmacology, the pharmacokinetics describe all the steps taken by any drug (pharmaceutical or radiopharmaceutical) to be delivered to the sites of action since the moment of administration. These steps are: absorption from the locale of administration to the bloodstream, distribution by blood (serum, blood cells and proteins), transport across cellular membranes to reach the sites of action, to be metabolized and finally excreted. With the radiotracers in use for brain imaging there is never absorption, because they are directly deposited in the bloodstream through an intravenous injection. However, when an iodine-labelled tracer ($^{123}$I-IMP, $^{123}$I-IBZM) is used, there is a need to block the thyroid, reducing radiation exposure. This is achieved by the oral administration of Lugol solution, iodide or iodate salts. All the other steps of the pharmacokinetic chain are present for either perfusion ($^{99m}$Tc-HMPAO) or neuroreceptor ligands ($^{123}$I-IBZM) in use nowadays. After their intravenous administration they have (1) to be delivered to the brain, according to the blood flow through the supplying arterial system, (2) to cross the blood–brain barrier, (3) to bind to either specific or non-specific cellular sites. In addition, they may (4) be metabolized either in neurons or elsewhere, and (5) are excreted through the hepatobiliary and renal pathways.

## Blood supply

It is provided by two main pairs of arteries, the internal carotids (right and left) branches of the common carotids, and the vertebral arteries, branches of the brachiocephalic arch and subclavian artery respectively on the right and left sides of the neck. Variants from this normal pattern of origin of the main arteries to the brain are of minor clinical importance. Much more relevant is the knowledge of the topographic distribution of the brain territories mainly supplied by each of the internal carotid and vertebral branches. Several anastomoses between the external carotid and

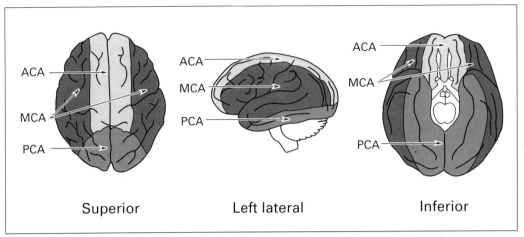

*Fig. 1. Representation of the vascular supply territories of the three main cerebral arteries*
*(ACA = anterior; MCA = middle; PCA = posterior)*

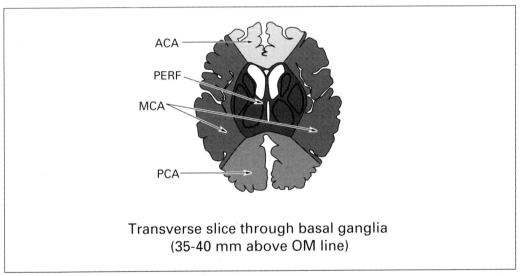

*Fig. 2. Vascular supply of the basal ganglia and thalamus is made via the perforating branches (PERF)*
*of the carotid and vertebrobasilar systems.*

the internal carotid, between the external carotid and the vertebrobasilar system, as well as between right and left internal carotid branches play an important role in the prognosis of neurological sequelae and surgical treatment of certain pathological conditions[2,4].

The terminal branches of the internal carotid artery are two for each hemisphere, the anterior, and the middle cerebral arteries. They supply the anterior, lateral and superior areas of the brain, whilst the posterior cerebral artery, a branch of the vertebrobasilar system, supplies the posterior and inferior areas of the cortex (Fig. 1).

Perforating branches of the carotid and vertebrobasilar systems supply the deeper nuclei, basal ganglia and thalamus (Fig. 2).

The anterior cerebral artery supplies the entire anterior two-thirds of the medial aspect of the cerebral hemispheres, including the corpus callosum, cingulate gyrus and superior frontal gyrus. The right and left anterior cerebral arteries communicate with each other through the anterior communicating artery, closing the anterior part of circle of Willis, just above the optic chiasm.

The middle cerebral artery supplies the cortex of the majority of the lateral surface of the cerebral hemispheres (frontal, parietal, temporal and occipital lobes), the insular and opercular surfaces, the lateral area of the orbital surface of the frontal lobe, the anterior temporal pole, and the lateral temporal cortex (upper two-thirds).

The posterior cerebral artery supplies the posterior areas of the cerebral hemispheres (cortical branches mainly to the visual cortex), thalamus, midbrain (central branches to the brainstem), choroid plexus and walls of the lateral and third ventricles (ventricular branches to the choroid plexus).

The smaller branches of each one of these three main arteries show multiple variations involving size, calibre, origin and short segments of duplication or island formation, rarely of clinical significance, except when they are associated with aneurysm formation. Even in the event of pathological occlusion of one important artery there are multiple permanent collaterals and others opening *de novo* to repair the injured territory. The circle of Willis[15] is the most classical of these collateral systems. It allows a theoretical communication between the anterior and posterior circulations through the posterior communicating arteries and between the right and left hemispheres through the anterior communicating artery. Although not functioning as a true equalizer or distributor of cerebral blood flow, the circle of Willis, if not patent (hypoplasia of one of the communicating arteries), may play an important role with adverse pathological consequences when one of the major arteries is diseased.

Other possible collateral systems include carotid-basilar connections (trigeminal artery, otic artery, and hypoglossal artery) other than the posterior communicating artery, carotid-vertebral connections (proatlantal and cervical intersegmental arteries), external carotid to vertebrobasilar communication via the occipital artery, leptomeningeal connections (the most frequent supratentorial being between the anterior and middle, and between the middle and posterior cerebral arteries), and finally other external-internal carotid arteries, connections via the ophthalmic artery and meningeal arteries.

A complicated network of capillaries carries the blood via the venous drainage system (pial veins) to the sinuses allowing the blood to return to the heart through the jugular veins. An important role of the cerebral venous system seems to be the control of total cerebral blood volume[1].

Both the arterial and venous systems are intimately related to the development of cerebral ischaemia, as well as the delivery of radioactive tracers mapping cerebral blood flow, metabolism and neuroreceptor availability.

The main mechanisms of ischaemia are global and focal. The former may be permanent or transient and the latter arterial, venous or arteriolar. In each case, the following changes can be identified during the early phases of cerebral ischaemic lesions: (1) neurons show various changes in volume and staining characteristics, (2) the nuclei of astrocytes are hypertrophic with hyperplasia, and (3) there is vacuolation of the neuropil. The different way of responding to an ischaemic insult by the neurons and astrocytes has been documented by several authors who are unanimous in considering neurons the most vulnerable elements to the effects of ischaemia[10] whilst astrocytes are the most resistant structures, with oligodendrocytes and myelin sheaths having an intermediate degree of vulnerability. In addition to these cellular changes, capillaries in areas of brain ischaemia show important abnormalities that may be directly implicated in the induction of local ischaemia. These comprise mechanical obstruction of the lumen, extrinsic mechanical compression, swelling of endothelial cells, spasms and modifications of the transendothelial transport of molecules or solutes.

Abnormalities of the blood–brain barrier (BBB) are evident and play an important role in the progression of the ischaemic insult. Structural changes in capillaries and arterioles reflected in transient alterations of the BBB to macromolecules remain to be characterized[6,23].

Before the description of the BBB and its properties, it is imperative to briefly discuss the cerebral blood flow – metabolism coupling and the factors inducing its alterations.

**Cerebral blood flow adaptation to physiology and disease**

The cerebral vascular network is not a system of rigid branching pipes. Regional cerebral blood flow (rCBF) depends on the perfusion pressure, the pressure difference between the inflow (arterial) and outflow (venous) pressures, and many other factors. Blood is a non-Newtonian fluid with a non-laminar flow pattern, the area of the cerebral vascular bed is not constant (significant variations occur in physiological and particularly disease states), the inflow perfusion pressure is pulsatile and the vessels actively change their calibre and may respond passively to changes from the inside or outside pressures over the walls.

The perfusion pressure seems to be one of the most important factors regulating the rCBF, so much so that reduction of perfusion pressure due to an increase in intracranial pressure is better tolerated than the drop of arterial pressure caused by haemorrhage[12,13]. In his experiments, Miller and co-workers[12] showed that CBF began to fall at 40 and 60 mmHg, respectively, with increased intracranial pressure and in response to haemorrhage. Several mechanisms have been described for this autoregulation of the CBF in general and rCBF in each particular area of the central nervous system. Regardless of these the important message is that in patients with areas of brain damage and oedema, drop in blood pressure must be avoided and the cerebral perfusion pressure kept at an optimal level. Increasing the arterial pressure is a severe mistake because it will not necessarily produce an increase in rCBF in the areas of brain damage, but oedema with a rise in the intracranial pressure and either no change or even drop in perfusion pressure.

Although both the perfusion pressure and resistance of the cerebrovascular network are important, other factors influencing the rCBF cannot be forgotten. Blood viscosity is one of them, directly dependent on the haematocrit, as well as gamma globulin and fibrinogen contents of the plasma proteins. Blood viscosity rises exponentially with their increase, and consequently rCBF decreases[20]. It is not rare for flow to stop and restart in the cerebral microcirculation. Apparently the force needed to restart flow is directly dependent on the haematocrit[14]. Autoregulation of CBF compensates for changes in blood viscosity. Patients with chronic obstructive airways disease (COAD) – (chronic bronchitis and emphysema) have high haematocrit stimulated by chronic hypoxia and their CBF, as measured with the multiprobe $^{133}$Xe method, is within normal limits[22].

Autoregulation maintains rCBF relatively constant, despite variations in the flow-influencing factors. The radionuclide methodology (multiprobe $^{133}$Xe) has demonstrated the normal CBF to be about 50 ml/100 g/min, decreasing slightly with increasing age.

There are only limited reserves of glucose and glycogen available in the brain (astrocytes), constantly dependent on blood supply to provide oxygen and glucose. Within a few minutes (not more than 7 min) neuronal tissue ATP drops to zero if oxygen supply is interrupted[17]. This points to a very intimate relationship between CBF and neuronal metabolism, usually said to be coupled. The average rate of glucose consumption is calculated at approximately 25 µM/100 g/min, very close to the average CBF. In physiological conditions any variation in the metabolic rates induces a CBF variation of similar amplitude and direction.

For instance, CBF increases with an acute increase in the arterial $pCO_2$. This is apparent by 2 min and reaches equilibrium within 12 min. Chronic adaptation is achieved in COAD patients with chronically elevated $pCO_2$. Changes in arterial $pO_2$ do not evoke significant changes in CBF. However, when there is impairment of the cerebrovascular response to arterial concentrations of $CO_2$, responses to hypoxia and to increases of the arterial concentration of $O_2$ are also impaired.

In summary, the vascular cerebral bed is reactive to arterial concentrations of $CO_2$, as well as to ionic changes ($Ca^{2+}$, $K^+$), adenosine concentration in the extracellular fluid, and neuropeptides. All of them may be used for pharmacological challenges of rCBF and neuronal metabolism.

## Blood–brain barrier

The blood–brain barrier (BBB) is the interface between the cerebral capillary circulation and the central nervous system tissue. Ehrlich in 1857[7] was the first to describe observations revealing this barrier phenomenon. He found that after the systemic administration of vital dyes, all organs were stained with the exception of the central nervous system (brain and spinal cord). A few years later another German scientist[8,9] made two important contributions to the history of the BBB. In his first paper, Goldmann[8] demonstrated, similarly to Ehrlich[7], that trypan blue did not stain the central nervous system after intravenous administration, whilst all the other tissues were coloured by the dye. In the second experiment[9] he observed that after the administration of trypan blue into the cerebrospinal fluid, the central nervous system was profusely stained. Since then long controversies about the anatomical configuration of the BBB have been perpetuated. Nowadays, the majority of the neuroscientists and neurophysiologists dedicated to the study of the BBB accept that the special characteristics of the cerebral endothelium are enough to support the idea of this tight endothelium[5] being the major anatomic component of the BBB. These characteristics are: (1) it is a sheet of cells connected by tight junctions and lying on a basement membrane; (2) its permeability to ions and hydrophilic compounds is very low; (3) it has a very low hydraulic conductance; (4) its intercellular junctions permit some solutes to have passive diffusion; (5) it has facilitated transport mechanisms for certain organic solutes; (6) it is possessed of saturation kinetics, stereospecificity and competitive interactions; (7) it contains induction mechanisms; (8) it has a high electrical resistance; (9) its permeability is increased by high osmolality values; and (10) it has a $Na^+$-$K^+$ pump located in the abluminal endothelial membrane.

How and why the capillaries of the central nervous system are so special, anatomically and functionally different from the ones in the other tissues, remains to be fully understood. However, recent reports gave evidence for a direct influence of the brain tissue over the cerebral endothelium and its properties. First, Stewart & Wiley in 1981[19] showed that when avascular brain tissue from 3-day-old quails is transplanted into the coelomic cavity of chick embryos, the chick endothelial cells vascularizing the brain grafts develop characteristics of a tight endothelium and form a competent blood–brain barrier. If, on the other hand, avascular embryonic quail coelomic grafts were transplanted into embryonic chick brain, the endothelial cells invading the mesenchymal tissue grafts in the chick brain gained the characteristics of a leaky endothelium at the capillary and venule level. Six years later, in 1987 Janzer & Raff[11] provided direct evidence that astrocytes (but not meningeal cells or fibroblasts) are capable of inducing BBB properties in non-neural endothelial cells *in vivo*.

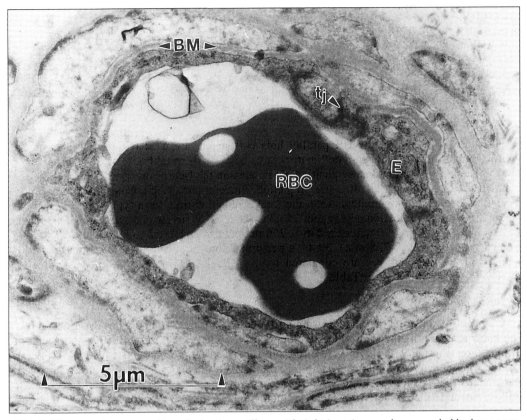

*Fig. 3. Electron microscopy slice of a brain capillary with tight junctions and surrounded by basement membrane and astrocytes. E = endothelial cell; Rbc = red blood cells, bm = basement membrane; tj = tight junction. (From R.F. Moss, St George's Hospital Medical School, London, UK.)*

Ultimately we can say that the blood in the capillary lumen is separated from the neurons by an effective barrier composed of the endothelial cells with tight junctions between them, and their basement membrane surrounded by multiple astrocytic processes (Fig. 3). This complex structure regulates the passage of solutes, nutrients and other chemicals transported in the blood from the capillary lumen to the neurons.

The intact BBB is not permeable to large molecules[16]. However, gases, water, glucose, electrolytes and amino acids can more or less easily pass through this barrier to reach the neurons and the small volume of extracellular space. Several mechanisms preside over this passage through the BBB. Water and gases cross via passive diffusion, whilst glucose and amino acids use transporter mechanisms with different energy expenditure.

Trauma, inflammatory processes and/or cerebrovascular insults may cause rupture of the blood–brain barrier with consequent disorganization of its characteristics of a tight endothelium. Therefore, intra- and extracellular concentrations of water, electrolytes and proteins may change significantly. Such a breakdown in the BBB enables molecules and compounds to leak from the blood into the extracellular space. Until the late 1970s this has been the major mechanism by which non-diffusible radiotracers ([99m]Tc-pertechnetate, [99m]Tc-GH, [99m]Tc-DTPA) were used to diagnose intracerebral primary or secondary tumours, as well as brain infarcts. Since the early 1980s lipophilic and neutral compounds ([123]I-IMP, [123]I-HIPDM, [99m]Tc-HMPAO, [99m]Tc-ECD,

[99mTc]-MRP 20) have emerged able to cross the intact BBB and to be retained in the brain, with consequent impact in the routine clinical practice of nuclear medicine. Nuclear neurology and psychiatry were giving the first steps towards a promising future.

**Neurotransmission**

The previous paragraphs have demonstrated the important role of cell-to-cell interaction in the central nervous system, particularly in respect to the influence of astrocytes over the endothelial characteristics. It appears that astrocytes may induce and maintain the particular characteristics of the cerebral tight endothelium. In addition, they may produce the necessary communication between neurons and capillaries in order to regulate local perfusion/blood flow and/or endothelial permeability, according to neuronal activity[3]. The mediators of this cell-to-cell interaction are unknown[11].

Beyond the BBB, cell-to-cell interactions are mainly between neurons. The space between two neurons is called the synaptic connection or cleft and is almost a virtual space filled in by neurotransmitters travelling from the pre-synaptic neuron to the post-synaptic cell and vice versa. The neuronal circuitry is made much more of chemical exchanges between neurons than simple electrical excitation or inhibition.

For the neurotransmission to take place several steps need to be considered: the synthesis of the neurotransmitter in the pre-synaptic neuron, its kinetics through the terminal axon to be released into the synapsis, the activation of post-synaptic receptors and the neurotransmitter metabolism, usually enzymatic and/or by pre-synaptic neuronal re-uptake. Any interference with one of these steps will obviously change the neurotransmission.

Nowadays there are multiple chemicals known to work as neurotransmitters, some of them as follows: γ-aminobutyric acid (GABA), acetylcholine (ACh), dopamine, noradrenaline, adrenaline, 5-hydroxytryptamine (5-HT), histamine (H), in addition to a number of amino acids and peptides. Very recently[18] nitric oxide (NO) and carbon monoxide (CO) have been reported to be serious candidates for a new class of atypical neurotransmitter-like neuronal messengers. NO mimics the effects of physiological nerve stimulation and is a mediator of blood vessel relaxation.

To complicate the system, for each neurotransmitter there are already multiple post-synaptic receptor sites recognized. For instance, $GABA_A$ and $GABA_B$; dopamine $D_1$, $D_2$, $D_3$, $D_4$; H1 and H2; 5-HT1A, 5-HT1B, 5-HT1C, 5-HT2, 5-HT3; muscarinic (M1, M2, M3) and nicotinic receptors for ACh; alpha and beta with subtypes for noradrenaline and adrenaline, are all identified and have been related to multiple neuropsychiatric diseases.

A wide range of agonist and/or antagonists of these neuroreceptors have been labelled with radiotracers, either positron ([11C], [18F]) or single photon emitters ([123I]) and appear in the literature as ligands for the investigation of patients with several neuropsychiatric diseases[21].

The addition of ligands working as precursors, at the level of the pre-synaptic neurons will improve our knowledge of neurotransmission, particularly in diseases, such as Parkinson and related parkinsonian syndromes. These will be more extensively discussed in Chapters 3 and 6 by respectively Verhoeff and Mazière.

**References**

1.  Auer, L.M., Oberbauer, R.W. & Schalk, H.V. (1983): Human pial vascular reactions to intravenous nimodipine infusion during EC–IC bypass surgery. *Stroke* **14**, 210–213.

2.     Baptista, A.G. (1963): Studies on the arteries of the brain. II. The anterior cerebral artery: some anatomic features and their clinical implications. *Neurology* **13**, 825–835.

3.     Bradbury, M.W.B. (1985): The blood–brain barrier. Transport across the cerebral endothelium. *Circ. Res.* **57(2)**, 213–222.

4.     Countee, R.W. & Vijayanathan, T. (1979): External carotid artery in internal carotid artery occlusion: angiographic, therapeutic, and prognostic considerations. *Stroke* **10**, 450–460.

5.     Crone, C. (1981): Tight and leaky endothelia. In: *Water transport across endothelia*, eds. H. Ussing, N. Bindslev, N.A. Lassen & O. Sten-Knudsen, pp. 256–267. Copenhagen: Munksgaard.

6.     DiChiro, G., Timins, E.L., Jones, A.E., Johnston, G.S., Hammock, M.K. & Swann, S.J. (1974): Radionuclide scanning and microangiography of evolving and completed brain infarction: a correlative study in monkeys. *Neurology* **24**, 418–423.

7.     Ehrlich, P. (1885): *Das Sauerstoff-Bederfuis des Organismus: eine farbenalytische Studie*. Berlin: Hirschward.

8.     Goldmann, E.E. (1909): Die aussere ind innere Sekretion des gesunden und kranken Organismus im Lichte der 'vitalen Farbung'. *Beitr. Klin. Chirurg.* **64**, 192–265.

9.     Goldmann, E.E. (1913): Vitalfarbung am Zentralnervensystem. *Abh. Preuss. Akad. Wiss. Phys. Math. Kl.* **1**, 1–60.

10.    Garcia, J.H. (1983): Ischaemic injuries of the brain: morphologic evolution. *Arch. Pathol. Lab. Med.* **107**, 157–161.

11.    Janzer, R.C. & Raff, M.C. (1987): Astrocytes induce blood–brain barrier properties in endothelial cells. *Nature* **325**, 253–257.

12.    Miller, J.D., Stanek, A.E. & Langfitt, T.W. (1972): Concepts of cerebral perfusion pressure and vascular compression during intracranial hypertension. *Prog. Brain Res.* **35**, 411–432.

13.    Miller, J.D., Stanek, A.E. & Langfitt, T.W. (1973): Cerebral blood flow regulation during experimental brain compression. *J. Neurosurg*, **39**, 186–196.

14.    Miller, J.D. & Bell, B.A. (1987): Cerebral blood flow variations with perfusion pressure and metabolism. In: *Cerebral blood flow. Physiologic and clinical aspects*, ed. J.H. Wood, pp. 19–130. New York: McGraw Hill.

15.    Pallie, W. & Samarasinghe, D.D. (1962): A study in the qualification of the circle of Willis. *Brain* **85**, 569–578.

16.    Reese, T.S. & Karnovsky, M.J. (1967): Fine structural localisation of a blood–brain barrier to exogenous peroxidase. *J. Cell. Biol.* **34**, 207–217.

17.    Siesjo, B.K. (1984): Cerebral circulation and metabolism. *J. Neurosurg.*, **60**, 883–908.

18.    Snyder, S.H. (1992): Nitric oxide: first in a new class of neurotransmitters? *Science* **257**, 494–496.

19.    Stewart, P.A. & Wiley, M.J. (1981): Developing nervous tissue induces formation of blood–brain barrier characteristics in invading endothelial cells: a study using quail-chick transplantation chimeras. *Dev. Biol.* **84**, 183–192.

20.    Thomas, D.J. (1982): Whole blood viscosity and cerebral blood flow. *Stroke* **13**, 285–287.

21.    Verhoeff, N.P.L.G. (1991): Pharmacological implications for neuroreceptor imaging. *Eur. J. Nucl. Med.* **18(7)**, 482–502.

22.    Wade, J.P.H. (1983): Transport of oxygen to the brain in patients with elevated haematocrit values before and after venesection. *Brain* **106**, 513–523.

23.    Wilmes, F.J., Garcia, J.H. & Conger, K.A. (1983): Mechanisms of blood–brain barrier breakdown after microembolization of the cat's brain. *J. Neuropathol. Exp. Neurol.* **42**, 421–438.

*New Trends in Nuclear Neurology and Psychiatry*, edited by D.C. Costa, G.F. Morgan and N. A. Lassen
© 1993 John Libbey & Company Ltd., pp. 25–36

# Chapter 3

# Imaging neurotransmission and neuroreceptors – physiological and pharmacological basis

N.P.L.G. Verhoeff

*Department of Nuclear Medicine, Academic Medical Centre, Meibergdreef 9, 1105 AZ Amsterdam Zuidoost (NH), The Netherlands*

Nowadays, information regarding neurotransmission in the human brain can be obtained *in vivo* using single photon emission tomography (SPET) or positron emission tomography (PET). Data from those studies (images) can be analysed using pharmacokinetic models. Several of those models are discussed for semiquantification or absolute quantification *in vivo* of parameters (binding potential, density and affinity) describing the neuroreceptor status in the brain. These models vary in their level of complexity, precision and accuracy. The data on the images are related to the underlying pharmacology of the neuroreceptor in a complex way, and therefore caution should be exercised when these models are used for drawing conclusions regarding possible implications on the pathophysiology of neuropsychiatric diseases.

## Introduction

The emphasis in imaging of neurotransmission is mainly on imaging of neuroreceptors as currently most tracers have been developed for that purpose[27–29,41,42]. Neuroreceptors are proteins in the membrane of neurons on which neurotransmitters, substances that can transmit signals from one nerve cell to another, can bind specifically just as a key fits into a lock. Often the lock, that is the receptor, can be opened by different keys and generally the door, that is the signal transduction system, has several different locks. Once the door is opened, the signal can go from outside the neuron to its interior. There may be more doors leading towards the room (the inner part of the neuron) and every door may lead to different signal pathways which may also interact with each other.

Single photon emission tomography (SPET) or positron emission tomography (PET) images using receptor specific tracers are quite different from those using perfusion tracers. Fig. 1 shows an $^{99m}$Tc-HMPAO SPET. Fig. 2 reveals SPET using the dopamine $D_2$ receptor specific tracer [$^{123}$I]-iodobenzamide ($^{123}$I-IBZM). In contrast to Fig. 1, the striatum in the centre having the highest density of $D_2$ receptors, is the most active.

## Semiquantification using ratios

In addition to neuroreceptor imaging it is important to develop a model for quantification of receptor affinity ($1/K_d$) and receptor density ($B_{max}$). As the application of PET models is complex

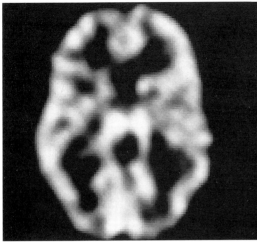

*Fig. 1. Brain perfusion SPET with $^{99m}Tc$-HMPAO in a 20-year-old male healthy volunteer, taken at 40 min p.i., 4 cm above and parallel to the canto-meatal line (5 min. slice, 1.2 cm/slice, 1 cm spacing).*

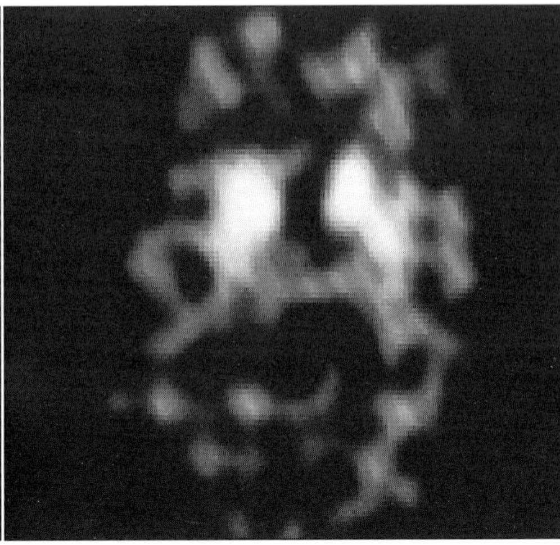

*Fig. 2. Dopamine $D_2$ receptor SPET with $^{123}I$-io-dobenzamide in a 19-year-old male healthy volun-teer, taken at 150 min. p.i., 4 cm above and parallel to the canto-meatal line (5 min/slice, 1.2 cm/slice, 1 cm spacing).*

and requires repeat studies in the same patient[26–29], there is an increasing willingness to obtain information from a single static single slice or multislice study. Assessment of group discrim-ination for clinical purposes does not necessarily benefit from the methods of optimization of parameters traditionally used in absolute quantification with PET[38]. Kinetic models requiring many estimated parameters may result in a large variation of the final parameters of interest. Repeated studies are inevitably accompanied by a larger radiation dose exposure of the subjects involved.

Ideally, quantification is absolute but may be relative, e.g. a ratio of a brain region with many receptors in the numerator and a brain region with few or no receptors in the denominator as background value. The regions are chosen based on the known receptor distribution from post-mortem studies. The distribution of the radioactive tracer in the brain changes with time p.i. For example $^{123}I$-IBZM reaches an equilibrium at about 1.5 h p.i. Subsequently the ratio of the region with many receptors (striatum) to the regions with only few receptors (cerebellum or cerebral cortex) remains constant for about 1 h, but decreases thereafter (Figs. 3 and 4). This is sufficient time for imaging *in vivo* with SPET.

Applying ratios is a common procedure in SPET with $^{123}I$-IBZM[3,36] or $^{123}I$-iodolisuride[4]. The use of ratios has also been validated for clinical purposes by comparison with parameters for the striatal $D_2$ receptor binding potential (i.e. the ratio $B_{max}/K_d$ according to Mintun *et al.* [32]) derived from compartment models in PET[5,23,45]. To estimate the striatal D2 receptor binding potential with SPET in parkinsonian patients, the cerebellum[4], the frontal cortex[3,36], and the occipital cortex[40] have all been used as denominators in the ratio as estimations of the 'free plus nonspe-cifically bound' ligand concentration.

Problems with the ratio method are:

(1) Receptor density and receptor affinity cannot be estimated separately. Only the 'binding potential', a combination of both, is obtained;

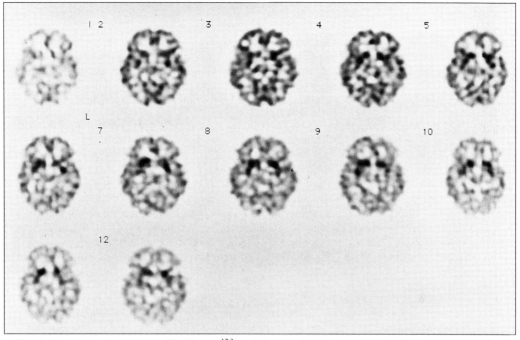

*Fig. 3. Dopamine D₂ receptor SPET with $^{123}$I-iodobenzamide in a 45-year-old female healthy volunteer, taken from 0–60 min p.i. at level 4 cm above canto-meatal line (5 min/slice, 1.2 cm/slice, no spacing). Slices normalized for global maximum.*

(2) The ratio may become 'contaminated' if a metabolite of the radio ligand with a different receptor affinity is formed in a substantial amount and crosses the blood–brain barrier (BBB);

(3) The non-specific binding of the reference region may be different from the region with a high receptor density;

(4) The non-specific binding of the reference region may be very low resulting in a large variability of the measured value from the image, thus allowing a large variability in the ratio values as well.

Advantages of the ratio method, if the last two issues above are not important, are:

(1) It provides a simple and rapid semi-quantification suitable for clinical use;

(2) It is less labour-intensive;

(3) It is less invasive as no blood samples have to be drawn by arterial lines;

(4) It is closer to the actually acquired image data and less dependent on the model assumed and the chosen parameters.

Some parameters have to be 'fixed' before they are used in the model. If the fixed values are not derived from a similar patient group, interpretation of the results from the model becomes more difficult. For example, the apparent systemic discrepancy between the maximal dopamine D₂ receptor density in the same human striatum measured *in vivo* with PET when two different tracers were used ([$^{11}$C]-raclopride and [$^{11}$C]-N-methylspiperone), may have been due to the fact that for the [$^{11}$C]-N-methylspiperone model a fixed dissociation rate constant of haloperidol was used based on measurements in living rats[46]. This was not used in the model for [$^{11}$C]-raclopride. It may well be that this fixed value was not applicable to the human subjects investigated.

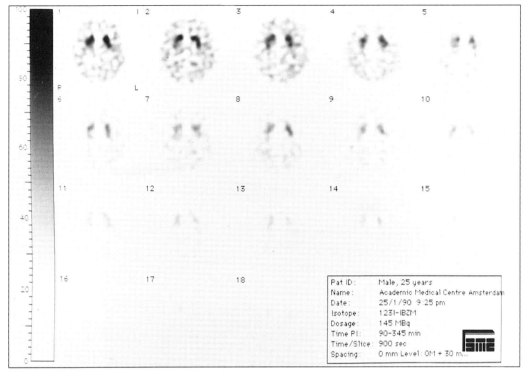

*Fig. 4. Dopamine D₂ receptor SPET with $^{123}$I-iodobenzamide in a 25-year-old male healthy volunteer, taken from 90–345 min p.i. at level 4 cm above the canto-meatal line (15 min slice, 1.2 cm/slice, no spacing). Slices normalized for global maximum.*

**Absolute quantification using various models**

To base an estimation of receptor density on a single image in time has drawbacks. To measure the affinity and density of receptors separately requires two studies using different specific activities (in MBq/nmol) of the radioligand. Several models used will now be discussed subsequently.

*Kinetic compartmental modelling*

A change in receptor affinity can only be discriminated from a change in receptor density when dynamic (kinetic) studies are performed. In the kinetic method, the pharmacodynamic behaviour of the tracer is modelled as transport between compartments, and measured values of tracer concentration in brain tissue and plasma over time are fit to equations derived from the model[18]. The kinetic approach follows the general model developed by Frost *et al.* for opiate receptor quantification with PET and [$^{11}$C]carfentanil[9] or [$^{11}$C]diprenorphine[35]. Briefly, tracer kinetics are modelled in three compartments as shown below:

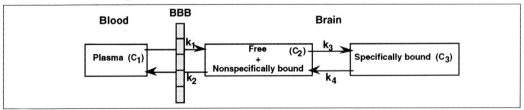

With the parameters in the following units:

$C_1$, $C_2$ and $C_3$ = tracer concentrations within compartments, in nM

$K_1 = \text{Flow} \times (1 - e^{-f1PS/Flow})$, in $\text{ml/min}_{-1} \times \text{g}^{-1}$;

$k_2$, $k_3$ and $k_4$ = passage constants between compartments, in $\text{min}^{-1}$.

For the additional parameters, which will be discussed later:

F = concentration of free ligand in the brain, in nM;
B = concentration of tracer specifically bound to receptor, in nM;
$k_{on}$ = bimolecular association rate constant ($\text{nM}^{-1} \times \text{min}^{-1}$);
$k_{off}$ = unimolecular dissociation rate constant ($\text{min}^{-1}$);
$f_1$ = free fraction in blood (blood free/$C_1$);
$f_2$ = free fraction in brain (brain free/$C_2$).

The model is defined by a set of differential equations describing the change in concentrations in the two brain compartments with time. With negligible receptor occupancy, these equations can be solved by analytical methods; complete derivations for the equations can be found in the work of Frost *et al.*[9] and Sadzot *et al.*[35]. At high specific activity, where receptor occupancy is negligible (B << $B_{max}$), the binding potential is related to the model parameters by the equation:

$$\text{Binding potential} = \frac{k_1 \times k_3}{f_1 \times k_2 \times k_4}$$

In dynamic saturation studies differing specific activities of the ligand involved are used[2,7]. In dynamic competition studies an *in vivo* displacement of the radioactive ligand from the brain by at least a 100-fold excess of competitive cold ligand is used[39] at a suitable moment after injection when there is known to be substantial specific binding to the receptor. From this *in vivo* displacement the dissociation rate constant $k_{off}$ can be determined. When a specific and a nonspecific area in the brain can be defined, an association rate constant $k_{on}$ can be obtained. The quotient of both will enable the determination of the equilibrium dissociation constant ($K_d$). The parameters can be displayed on a pixel-by-pixel basis[2].

With a simplified approach using two-compartmental analysis, radioligand delivery (perfusion dependent) and distribution volume (receptor binding capacity dependent) can be quantified separately, e.g. for CBZ receptors using [$^{11}$C]flumazenil and PET[10].

*Equilibrium imaging*

In the equilibrium approach, conditions are chosen so that the net transport between compartments is zero, and the relationships of concentrations in the measurable compartment(s) (i.e. plasma) are used to calculate the values. In one approach, taken by Farde *et al.*[6,7] to model the $D_2$ receptor tracer [$^{11}$C]raclopride, the experiment is carried out essentially as for the kinetic approach, and then brain and plasma time-activity curves are analysed to identify the point at which the function of bound activity B(t) peaks; at this point, dB/dt = 0 and a state of transient equilibrium exists. Disadvantages of this method are: (1) the entire data set needs to be collected, but only a subset of data is used; (2) identifying the range of times at which the approximation dB/dt = 0 is valid may be difficult; and (3) the concentration of free radioligand F is unknown and is assumed to be equal to that in a brain area devoid of receptors[2,6,7]. This assumption is not valid for most tracers, especially when labelled with $^{123}$I for SPET, since nonspecific binding is rarely negligible compared to free[41,42]. Nevertheless, a combination of the method of Farde *et al.*[6,7] to identify the peak time of B(t) and the ratio method for semiquantification of the binding potential may be useful for SPET studies as has been shown in the example of $D_2$ receptors[33].

*Constant infusion protocols*

Further absolute quantification of receptor density and affinity may be possible under real equilibrium conditions using constant infusion protocols as first described by Frey *et al.*[8] for [$^3$H]scopolamine and later elaborated by Lassen[22]. In this way, a steady state of tracer in the brain and plasma is achieved and the equilibrium condition is maintained over a long period of time. The length of time required to achieve equilibrium conditions can be reduced by administering an initial bolus, followed by constant infusion. For instance, using the opiate antagonist [$^{11}$C]cyclofoxy in a rat model, Kawai *et al.*[15] determined that with an appropriate ratio of bolus to infusion rate, equilibrium conditions could be reached within 45–90 min. Also, Laruelle *et al.*[21] used a similar protocol in a baboon where following an initial bolus injection, the radiotracer [$^{123}$I]iomazenil was infused at a constant rate for 5 to 8 h. The results of this constant infusion paradigm were very similar to those from a kinetic analysis. Moreover, by using different specific activities of the [$^{123}$I]iomazenil, Scatchard analysis was performed from the data obtained *in vivo*. The results were very similar to those from the membrane homogenates obtained from the animal under investigation after sacrifice[21].

At equilibrium, the concentration of receptor bound ligand ($B_e$) is given by:

$$B_e = \frac{B_{max} \times F}{K_d + F}$$

Rearrangement at high specific activity ($B_e \ll B_{max}$) provides:

$$\frac{B_e}{F} = \frac{B_{max} - B_e}{K_d} = \frac{B_{max}}{K_d} = \text{binding potential}$$

Thus, a single measurement of the concentration of receptor bound tracer ($B_e$) and free tracer (F) will give the binding potential. If equilibrium conditions are met, then the free level in the brain ($f_2 \times C_2$) will equal the free level in the plasma ($f_1 \times C_1$), and the specifically bound tracer can be derived from the total concentration measured by SPET ($C_{total}$) as follows:

$$\text{Given that } C_{total} = C_2 + C_3; C_3 = B_e \text{ ; and } f_1 \times C_1 = f_2 \times C_2$$

$$C_{total} = \frac{f_1 \times C_1}{f_2} + B_e; \text{ or } B_e = C_{total} - \frac{f_1 \times C_1}{f_2}$$

The plasma free fraction $f_1$ and concentration $C_1$ are measured directly. The free fraction in the brain, $f_2$, is taken from the mean value derived in kinetic experiments. However, the assumption that the free level in the brain ($f_2$) can be estimated directly by measurement of the free parent compound in the plasma needs to be validated.

At equilibrium, in principle, the binding potential can be calculated in any brain region, from a single SPET image and a single measurement of free parent radioligand concentration in blood. Because the activity in the brain is constant, the length of the image acquisition can be adjusted relative to the sensitivity of the SPET system to obtain reliable counting statistics with lower injected amounts of radioactivity. The constant infusion method might be easier to perform in humans than the kinetic method, which requires multiple scan acquisitions and arterial sampling. Arterial blood sampling would not be necessary, as under plasma steady state conditions, venous and arterial radiotracer concentrations equilibrate and plasma free parent compound could be measured in venous blood. The latter assumption also needs experimental confirmation, especially as eventually in clinical studies the $f_2$ fraction will be estimated on the basis of the free parent compound in venous plasma.

**Drawbacks of some models for absolute quantification**

Several drawbacks are present in some of these models when they are applied to the *in vivo* situation.

(a) Scatchard analysis requires more than 50 per cent occupancy of a binding site by a radioactive ligand to determine reliable parameters of the interaction of that site with the ligand[39]. Clearly, this is not feasible *in vivo* as tracer kinetic methods imply that there is no interference with the system that is actually being measured. Furthermore, the subjects investigated may suffer considerable side-effects. Thus, *in vivo* investigations often contain insufficient saturation curve data for Scatchard analysis.

(b) Hill plot analysis is a graphical transformation of saturation curve data with log [Free ligand] on the *x*-axis and log {[ per cent Ligand bound]/(100 – [ per cent Ligand bound]} on the *y*-axis. With independent binding to a site with one apparent affinity, the slope or Hill coefficient equals 1. A Hill coefficient > 1 indicates positive cooperativity, whereas a Hill coefficient < 1 indicates negative cooperativity or multiple binding sites. This type of analysis[39] requires for assessment of cooperativity the fractional occupancy of a binding site in a range from 2 per cent to 95 per cent. Thus, it may be difficult to obtain any information about cooperativity from *in vivo* studies.

(c) For Scatchard analysis and bimolecular kinetic studies it is often assumed that the reactions take place under pseudo-first order conditions. In this situation, only a small amount (< 10 per cent) of the radioligand added is assumed to be bound, so that the unbound concentration of drug almost equals the total amount of drug added[30]. *In vivo* it is likely that these assumptions cannot always be met in the brain if there is considerable brain retention, in particular in case of a rapid decline in tracer concentration in the blood. For example, about 10 per cent of the injected dose of [$^{123}$I]-iomazenil is taken up by the brain[41,43] and many tracers have high brain/blood ratios. The concentration of the tracer in the extracellular fluid directly surrounding surface membrane receptors is not known. If this concentration is low, ligand that has just dissociated from the receptor may be more inclined to bind to the majority of unbound receptors nearby[1].

(d) In bimolecular kinetic analysis the kinetic constants for the labelled ligand should be determined in separate experiments[30].

(e) In comparison of equilibrium binding studies of a radioligand with and without displacer and of bimolecular kinetic competition studies, the time needed to reach equilibrium is not only dependent on the $k_{on}$ and $k_{off}$ of the labelled ligand but also on the $k_{on}$ and $k_{off}$ of the unlabelled ligand. For saturation studies, this time is defined when at least 97 per cent of $B_e$ is measured. This requires an incubation of at least five half-lives, i.e. a period of at least $5 \times 0.698$/observed $k_{on}$ under pseudo-first order conditions. Thus, the unlabelled ligand may determine the time needed to reach equilibrium if its affinity is lower (i.e. a lower $k_{on}$) than that of the labelled ligand. For competition studies, this time is defined when at least 97 per cent of the final equilibrium value has been reached. This requires a period[30] of $1.75/k_{off}$. Thus, when the competing unlabelled ligand has a higher affinity (i.e. a lower $k_{off}$) than the radioligand, the time to reach equilibrium is dependent on the $k_{off}$ of the unlabelled ligand. The implication is that it may take a longer time for a study to reach equilibrium when a protocol is used with both unlabelled and labelled ligand than for a study which makes use of labelled ligand only.

(f) The assumption of an irreversible binding of the ligand to the receptor as in Patlak plot analysis[47,48] is only valid if the $k_{off}$ is negligible. Likewise, the assumption that nonspecific binding is irreversible, is constant or is a constant percentage of total binding over time may, in some cases, prove to be erroneous. In several studies it has been shown that specific binding of several ligands may be reversible and that nonspecific binding as a percentage of total binding can change (and decline) over time[7,41,44]. The latter is especially important for lipophilic iodinated tracers developed for neuroreceptor imaging in the brain, as generally the high membrane-buffer (or octanol-water) coefficient is accompanied by a high nonspecific binding to the lipid bilayer membrane[39].

(g) It is important which area in the brain is selected as representative for nonspecific binding. Problems resulting from too large a variability of the measured values for radioactivity in the reference region have been discussed above. The cerebellum may not always be a correct choice according to studies in rats[16,17] and humans[19].

(h) When attempts are made for absolute quantification, the partial volume effect of the imaging technique will have to be borne in mind since discrepancies in the estimation of specific versus nonspecific binding between SPET (and probably also PET) and other techniques for quantification are observed. For dopamine $D_2$ receptors striatum/cerebellum ratios have been obtained of 2.0 in humans with [$^{123}$I]iodolisuride SPET, whereas in a brain phantom[26] the corresponding ratio was 7.6. Similarly, the striatum/cerebral cortex ratios of approximately 2 obtained in baboons with [$^{123}$I]IBZM SPET increased to approximately 8 as measured with *ex vivo* autoradiography[12].

(i) It is generally assumed that the amount of radioactivity visualized *in vivo* is mainly a reflection of receptor density. However, for the CBZ receptor and the N receptor it has been reported that there may be different affinity states for the agonist [$^{11}$C]nicotine and antagonist [$^{11}$C]flumazenil respectively, potentially dependent on modulation by endogenous agonists[20,31,34]. This might also be the case for receptors when an excessive amount of endogenous agonist is present, as well as for $D_2$ receptors[13].

## Conclusion

The models presented for semiquantification and absolute quantification may be useful for clinical studies as long as one remains critical regarding the value of the resulting parameters. The value of the parameters may be expressed using clinical epidemiological measures of reliability such as precision, accuracy, inter-observer variability, sensitivity, specificity, and predictive value. Furthermore, one should be aware that neuroreceptor membrane proteins only play a limited role in neurotransmission besides many other components in the signal transduction chain such as G-proteins[11,14,24,25,37]. Taking these aspects into consideration, clinical studies using SPET or PET may indeed play a role in unravelling the pathophysiology of various neuropsychiatric disorders.

## Dictionary

**affinity** = strength of binding of a ligand to a receptor.
**agonist** = ligand exerting an effect on the cell after binding to its receptor.
**antagonist** = ligand exerting no effect on the cell after binding to its receptor, thus opposing the actions of the corresponding agonist binding to the same site.
**CBZ** = central benzodiazepine.
**cooperativity** = binding of one ligand to a site increases (positive cooperativity, uncommon) or decreases (negative cooperativity, common) the affinity of another ligand for the next unoccupied site.
**D** = dopamine.
**ligand** = (a) Pharmacology: specific chemical substance that conveys information for the regulation of intracellular processes and that acts both as messenger and as message through interac-

tion (forming a complex) with a specific receptor; (b) Nuclear medicine: an organic molecule that donates the necessary electrons to form coordinate covalent bonds with metallic ions.

**modulation** = the alteration of conformation of a receptor following interaction with a ligand (e.g. change in affinity for a ligand due to binding of an endogenous agonist at another site than where the ligand in question binds to the receptor).

**N** = nicotine.

**Patlak analysis** = a graphical transformation of an *in vivo* time curve with the time-integral of [Ligand concentration in the plasma] on the *x*-axis and [Specifically bound ligand] on the *y*-axis; from the slope the rate constant of binding of the ligand to the receptors from the plasma pool and the free and nonspecifically bound ligand ($k_3$) can be calculated; assuming there is no dissociation of the ligand from the receptor, $k_3$ is equal to the product of the association rate constant and the quantity of unoccupied receptors.

**receptor** = (a) generally: any cellular constituent that exhibits chemical specificity and that plays a key role in regulating the cellular effects of a particular active substance; (b) more specifically: surface binding sites that play simultaneously both a recognition and an activation role in terms of regulating cell function.

**Scatchard analysis** = graphical transformation of saturation curve data with [Bound ligand] on the *x*-axis and [Bound ligand]/[Free ligand] on the *y*-axis; in the case of one binding site a straight line results with $K_d = -1/\text{slope}$ and $B_{max}$ = the intercept on the *x*-axis; *in vivo* at least two points are needed to create the graph, obtained by injecting the radioligand with high and low specific activity in two separate experiments, and determining the parameters at equilibrium, when the curve for specific binding reaches a maximum.

**striatum** = caudate nucleus and putamen, together the components of the basal ganglia that receive most of the afferent input from other parts of the brain.

**transduction** = bringing over of a signal, a message, by molecular means, from one cell to another or within one cell; the starting and ending point of the signal transduction process can be non-molecular (e.g. electric, acoustic, visual, physical, tactile, thermal, consciousness) processes.

## Acknowledgements

The author thanks Prof. R.B. Innis, MD, PhD, and his co-workers at the Neurochemical Brain Imaging Department of Psychiatry, Yale University School of Medicine, West Haven, Connecticut, USA, regarding the provision of as yet unpublished recently acquired data, especially concerning the application of the constant infusion method for imaging central benzodiazepine receptors.

## References

1. Beer, H.F., Bläuenstein, P.A., Hasler, P.H., Delaloye, B., Riccabona, G., Bangerl, I., Hunkeler, W., Bonetti, E.P., Pieri, L., Richards, G.J. & Schibiger, P.A. (1990): *In vitro* and *in vivo* evaluation of iodine-123-ro 16-0154: a new imaging agent for SPECT investigations of benzodiazepine receptors. *J. Nucl. Med.* **31**, 1007–1014.

2. Blomqvist, G., Pauli, S., Farde, L., Eriksson, L., Persson, A. & Halldin, C. (1990): Maps of receptor binding parameters in the human brain – a kinetic analysis of PET measurements. *Eur. J. Nucl. Med.* **16**, 257–265.

3. Brücke, T., Podreka, I., Angelberger, P., Wenger, S., Topitz, A., Küfferle, B., Müller, C. & Deecke, L (1991): Dopamine D2 receptor imaging with SPECT: studies in different neuropsychiatric disorders. *J. Cereb. Blood Flow Metab.* **11**, 220–228.

4. Chabriat, H., Levasseur, M., Vidailhet, M., Loc'h, C., Mazière, B., Bourguignon, M.H., Bonnet, A.M., Raynaud, C., Agid, Y., Syrota, A. & Samson, Y. (1992): *In vivo* SPECT imaging of D2 receptor with iodine-iodolisuride: results in supranuclear palsy. *J. Nucl. Med.* **33**, 1481–1485.

5. Delforge, J., Loc'h, C., Hantraye, P. *et al.* (1991): Kinetic analysis of central [76]Br-bromolisuride binding to dopamine D2 receptors studied by PET. *J. Cereb. Blood Flow Metab.* **6**, 914–926.

6.  Farde, L., Eriksson, L., Blomqvist, G. & Halldin, C. (1989): Kinetic analysis of central [$^{11}$C]raclopride binding to D$_2$ dopamine receptors studied with PET: a comparison to the equilibrium analysis. *J. Cereb. Blood Flow Metab.* **9**, 696–708.

7.  Farde, L., Wiesel, F.A., Stone-Elander, S., Halldin, C., Nordström, A.L., Hall, H. & Sedvall, G.(1990): D$_2$ dopamine receptors in neuroleptic-naive schizophrenic patients. *Arch. Gen. Psychiat.ry* **47**, 213–219.

8.  Frey, K.A., Ehrenkaufer, R.L.E., Beaucage, S. & Agranoff, B.W. (1985): Quantitative *in vivo* receptor binding. I. Theory and application to the muscarinic cholinergic receptor. *J. Neurosci.* **5**, 421–428.

9.  Frost, J.J., Douglas, K.H., Mayber, H.S., Dannals, R.F., Links, J.M., Wilson, A.A., Ravert, H.T., Crozier, W.C. & Wagner, H.N. Jr. (1989): Multicompartmental analysis of [$^{11}$C]carfentanyl binding to opiate receptors in humans measured by positron emission tomography. *J. Cereb. Blood Flow Metab.* **9**, 398–409.

10. Holthoff, V.A., Koeppe, R.A., Frey, K.A., Paradise, A.H. & Kuhl, D.E. (1991): Differentiation of radioligand delivery and binding in the brain: validation of a two-compartment model for [$^{11}$C]flumazenil. *J. Cereb. Blood Flow Metab.* **11**, 745–752.

11. Houslay, M.D. (1992): G-protein linked receptors: a family probed by molecular cloning and mutagenesis procedures. *Clin. Endocrinol.* **36**, 525–534.

12. Innis, R.B., Al-Tikriti, M., Woods, S.W., Zoghbi, S., Roth, R.H., Charney, D.S., Heninger, G.R., Smith, E.O., Zubal, I.G., Alavi, A., Hoffer, P.B. & Kung, H.F. (1990): SPECT imaging of the dopamine D2 receptor in primate brain. *J. Nucl. Med.* **31**, 883 (abstr.)

13. Innis, R.B., Malison, R.T., Al-Tikriti, M., Hoffer, P.B., Sybirska, E.H., Seibyl, J.P., Zoghbi, S.S., Baldwin, R.M. Laruelle, M., Smith, E.O., Charney, D.S., Heninger, G., Elsworth, J.D. & Roth, R.H. (1992): Amphetamine-stimulated dopamine release competes *in vivo* for [$^{123}$I]IBZM binding to the D$_2$ receptor in nonhuman primates. *Synapse* **10**, 177–184.

14. Johnson, G.L. & Dhanasekaran, N. (1989): The G-protein family and their interaction with receptors. *Endocr. Rev.* **10**, 317–331.

15. Kawai, R., Carson, R.E., Dunn, B., Newman, A.H., Rice, K.C. & Blasberg, R.G. (1991): Regional brain measurement of B$_{max}$ and $K_d$ with the opiate antagonist cyclofoxy: equilibrium studies in the conscious rat. *J. Cereb. Blood Flow Metab.* **11**, 529–544.

16. Kawai, R., Carson, R.E., Rice, K.C. & Blasberg, R.G. (1990): Evaluation of methods to determine nonspecific tissue binding on K$_d$ and B$_{max}$ estimates using the opiate receptor antagonist (–)-cyclofoxy [(–)CF] and equilibrium studies. *J. Nucl. Med.* **31**, 810 (abstr.)

17. Kawai, R., Channing, M., Newman, A.H. & Blasberg, R (1990): Nonspecific brain tissue binding of the opiate antagonist (–)cyclofoxy [(–)CF]: regional variation and time dependency. *J. Nucl. Med.* **31**, 883 (Abstract).

18. Kuikka, J.T., Bassingthwaighte, J.B., Henrich, M.M. & Feinendegen, L.E. (1991): Mathematical modelling in nuclear medicine. *Eur. J. Nucl. Med.* **18**, 351–362.

19. Lamoureux, G., Dupont, R.M., Gillin, J.C., Ashburn, W.L., Halpern, S.E., De Sherbrooke, U. & Quebec, P. (1990): A geomorphological description of the absolute uptake, cortical distribution and washout of $^{13}$I-iodoamphetamine (IMP) in a group of normal subjects. *Eur. J. Nucl. Med.* **16**, S144 (abstr.)

20. Larsson, C., Nilsson, L., Halen, A. & Nordberg, A. (1986): Subchronic treatment of rats with nicotine: effects on tolerance and on $^3$H-acetylcholine and $^3$H-nicotine binding in the brain. *Drug Alcohol Depend.* **17**, 37–45.

21. Laruelle, M., Abi-Dargham, A., Rattner, Z., Al-Tikriti, M.S., Zea-Ponce, Y., Zoghbi, S.S., Charney, D.S., Price, J., Frost, J.J., Hoffer, P.B., Baldwin, R.M. & Innis, R.B. (1993): SPECT measurement of benzodiazepine receptor number and affinity in primate brain: a constant infusion paradigm with [$^{123}$I]iomazenil. *Eur. J. Pharmacol.* in press.

22. Lassen, N.A. (1992): Neuroreceptor quantitation *in vivo* by the steady-state principle using constant infusion or bolus injection of radioactive tracers. *J. Cereb. Blood Flow Metab.* **12**, 709–716.

23. Leenders, K.L. (1986): Movement disorders. a study with positron emission tomography. Thesis. Free University, Amsterdam.

24. Linder, M.E. & Gilman, A.G. (1992): G-proteins. Tucked into the internal surface of the cell's outer membrane, these versatile molecules coordinate cellular reponses to a multitude of signals that impinge from without. *Sci. Am.* **July**, 36–43.

25. Manji, H.K. (1992): G-proteins: implications for psychiatry. *Am. J. Psychiatry* **149**, 746–760.

26. Mazière, B., Loc'h, C., Bourguignon, M., Chabriat, H., Raynaud, C., Levasseur, M. & Syrota, A. (1990): Imaging D$_2$ receptors with SPECT and $^{123}$I-iodolisuride. *Eur. J. Nucl. Med.* **16**, S112 (abstr.)

27. Mazière, B. & Mazière, M. (1990): Where have we got to with neuroreceptor mapping of the human brain? *Eur. J. Nucl. Med.* **16**, 817–835.

28. Mazière, B. & Mazière, M. (1991): Positron emission tomography studies of brain receptors. *Fundam. Clin. Pharmacol.* **5**, 61–91.

29. Mazière, B., Mazière, M., Delforge, J. & Syrota, A. (1991): Contribution of positron emission tomography to pharmacokinetic studies. In: *New trends in pharmacokinetics*, eds. A. Rescigno & A.K. Thakur, pp. 169–187. New York: Plenum Press.

30. McPherson, G.A. (1989): A mathematical approach to receptor characterization. In: *Receptor pharmacology and function*, eds. M. Williams, R.A. Glennon & P.B.M.W.M. Timmermans, pp. 47–84. New York: Marcel Dekker.

31. Miller, L.G., Greenblatt, D.J., Barnhill, J.G., Summer, W.R. & Shader, R.I. (1988): 'GABA shift' *in vivo* : enhancement of benzodiazepine binding *in vivo* by modulation of endogenous GABA. *Eur. J. Pharmacol.* **148**, 123–130.

32. Mintun, M.A., Raichle, M.E., Kilbourn, M.R., Wooten, G.F. & Welch, M.J. (1984): A quantitative model for the *in vivo* assessment of drug binding sites with positron emission tomography. *Ann. Neurol.* **15**, 217–227.

33. Pilowsky, L.S., Costa, D.C., Ell, P.J., Murray, R.M., Verhoeff, N.P.L.G. & Kerwin, R.W. (1992): Clozapine, single photon emission tomography, and the $D_2$ dopamine receptor blockade hypothesis of schizophrenia. *Lancet* **340**, 199–202.

34. Romanelli, L., Ohman, B., Adem, A. & Nordberg, A (1988): Subchronic treatment of rats with nicotine: interconversion of nicotinic receptor subtypes in brain. *Eur. J. Pharmacol.* **148**, 289–291.

35. Sazdot, B., Price, J.C., Mayberg, H.S., Douglass, K.H. Dannals, R.F., Lever, J.R., Ravert, H.T., Wilson, A.A., Wagner, H.N. Jr, Feldman, M.A. & Frost J.J. (1991): Quantification of human opiate receptor concentration and affinity using high and low specific activity [[11]C]diprenorphine and positron emission tomography. *J. Cereb. Blood Flow Metab.* **11**, 204–219.

36. Schwarz, J., Tatsch, K., Arnold, G., Gasser, T., Trenkwalder, C., Kirsch, C.M. & Oertel, W.H. (1992): [123]I-iodobenzamide SPECT predicts dopaminergic responsiveness in patients with *de novo* parkinsonism. *Neurology* **42**, 556–561.

37. Spiegel, A.M., Shenker, A. & Weinstein, L.S. (1991): Receptor-effector coupling by G-proteins: implications for normal and abnormal signal transduction. *Endocr. Rev.* **13**, 536–565.

38. Strother, S.C., Liow, J.S., Moeller, J.R., Sidtis, J.J., Dhawan, V.J. & Rottenberg, D.A. (1991): Absolute quantification in neurological PET: do we need it? *J. Cereb. Blood Flow Metab.* **11** (Suppl 1), A3–A16.

39. Titeler, M. (1989): Receptor binding theory and methodology. In: *Receptor pharmacology and function*, eds. M. Williams, R.A. Glennon & P.B.M.W.M. Timmermans, pp. 1745. New York, Marcel Dekker.

40. Van Royen, E.A., Verhoeff, N.P.L.G., Speelman, J.D., Wolters, E.Ch.M.J., Kuiper, M.A. & Janssen, A.G.M. (1993): Diminished striatal dopamine $D_2$ receptor activity in multiple system atrophy and progressive supranuclear palsy demonstrated by [123]I-IBZM SPECT. *Arch. Neurol.* in press.

41. Verhoeff, N.P.L.G. (1993): Neuroreceptor ligand imaging by single photon emission computerised tomography (SPECT). Thesis. University of Amsterdam.

42. Verhoeff, N.P.L.G. (1991): Pharmacological implications for neuroreceptor imaging. *Eur. J. Nucl. Med.* **18**, 482–502.

43. Verhoeff, N.P.L.G., Van Royen, E.A., Overweg, J., Limburg, M., Hijdra, A. & Linszen, D. (1990): [123]I-iomazenil whole body distribution in human volunteers. *Eur. J. Nucl. Med.* **16**, 461 (abstr.)

44. Verhoeff, N.P.L.G., Costa, D.C., Ell, P.J., Toone, B., Palasidou, E., Cullum, I.D., Bobeldijk, M., Miller, R., Syed, G.M.S., Barrett, J.J., Soricelli, A. & Van Royen, E.A. (1991): Dopamine $D_2$-receptor imaging with dynamic [123]I-IBZM SPET in patients with schizophrenia or HIV encephalopathy. In: *Nuclear medicine. The state of the art of nuclear medicine in Europe.* eds. H.A.E. Schmidt & J.B. Van der Schoot. European Nuclear Medicine Congress Amsterdam, May 20–24, 1990. Stuttgart-New York: Schattauer. *Nucl. Med. Suppl* **27**, 207–212.

45. Wienhard, K., Coenen, H.H., Pawlik, G.,Rudolph, J., Laufer, P., Kovkar, S., Stöcklin, G. & Heiss, W.D. (1990): PET studies of dopamine receptor distribution using [[18]F]fluoroethylspiperone: findings in disorders related to the dopaminergic system. *J. Neural Transm.* **81**, 195–213.

46. Wong, D.F., Tune, L., Shaya, E., Pearlson, G., Yung, B., Dannals, R.F., Wilson, A.A., Ravert, H.T., Wagner, H.N. Jr & Gjedde A. (1992): The comparison of dopamine receptor density estimated by raclopride and NMSP in the same living human brain. *J. Nucl. Med.* **33**, 847 (abstr.)

47.     Wong, D.F., Wagner, H.N. Jr, Dannals, R.F., Links, J.M., Frost, J.J., Ravert, H.T., Wilson, A.A., Rosenbaum, A.E., Gjedde, A., Douglass, K.H., Petronis, J.D., Folstein, M.F., Tung, J.K.T., Burns, D. & Kuhar, M.J. (1984): Effects of age on dopamine and serotonin receptors measured by positron tomography in living human brain. *Science* **226**, 1393–1396.

48.     Wong, D.F., Wagner, H.N. Jr, Tune, L.E., Dannals, R.F., Pearlsson, G.D., Links, J.M., Tamminga, C.A., Broussole, E.P., Ravert, H.T., Wilson, A.A., Toung, J.K.T., Malat, J., Williams, J.A., O'Tuama, L.A., Snyder, S.H., Kuhar, M.J. & Gjedde, A. (1986): A positron emission tomography reveals elevated $D_2$ dopamine receptors in drug-naive schizophrenics. *Science* **234**, 1558–1563.

# Section III
# INSTRUMENTATION

The understanding of the characteristics of different instruments (either general purpose or dedicated tomographic cameras) available to carry out brain SPET is paramount for those who desire to obtain the best performance out of this evolving nuclear medicine technology.

In addition, quality assurance (QA) has to be carefully observed, particularly when quantitative analysis of any kind is to be performed.

*New Trends in Nuclear Neurology and Psychiatry*, edited by D.C. Costa, G.F. Morgan and N. A. Lassen
© 1993 John Libbey & Company Ltd., pp. 39–62

# Chapter 4

# Instrumentation for brain SPET: guidelines and quantification

P.H. Jarritt and K. Kouris

*Institute of Nuclear Medicine, University College of London Medical School, London, UK*

## Introduction

Whilst the technique of single photon emission tomography (SPET) was introduced by Kuhl & Edwards[26] as early as 1963 with a technological development concentrated on the brain, the subsequent development of instrumentation for brain SPET has followed the innovation of radiopharmaceuticals. Little instrument development has taken place in isolation from the available radiotracers. The development of devices for brain SPET imaging can be categorized by detector type. Firstly, those based upon multiple discrete detectors using collimation and detector motion to sample the volume of the brain. Examples of such systems are those first developed by Kuhl & Edwards[26] and more recently Strichman Medical Equipment[37] and Medimatic[38]. Secondly, there are systems based upon Anger logic for calculation of energy and position of a gamma photon interaction with a scintillation detector. Systems using a single Anger gamma camera for brain SPET are now being superseded by systems with two, three or four cameras. A further step in the optimization of this Anger type technology is the development of the annular position sensitive scintillation detector[11].

There are a number of factors which are common to all these developments. Particular emphasis has been placed on the optimization of patient position relative to the detector through changes in detector shape – circular detectors have been replaced by rectangular fields of view. These changes have been directed to minimizing contact with the patients' shoulders and hence enabling the detector(s) to approach nearer to the patients. The optimization of resolution and sensitivity has been of paramount importance. These developments have occurred through the improvement of collimators and detector configurations, some of which permit non-circular sampling trajectories.

This chapter was conceived from a desire to understand the elements of the tomographic process which impinge on image quality and quantification of brain SPET data and in particular which may lead to systematic variations in calculated values from system to system. It briefly reviews the status of the single Anger gamma camera system and compares this with the current development of multi-detector brain SPET systems. Performance characteristics of a number of systems are presented for comparative purposes. These are based both on experimental measurements by the authors and from publications in the refereed literature and manufacturers' specifications.

This is followed by a section on acquisition and processing protocols. Brain SPET now encompasses a range of clinical measurements including the measurement of brain blood flow using dynamic ($^{133}$Xe) and static ($^{99m}$Tc-HMPAO) radiopharmaceutical distributions. Measurements of breakdown in blood–brain barrier have been made using such tracers as $^{99m}$Tc-pertechnetate and $^{99m}$Tc-DTPA, measurements of blood volume using $^{99m}$Tc-red blood cells and more recently tumour markers such as $^{201}$Tl-chloride and receptor markers using a range of molecules labelled with either $^{99m}$Tc or $^{123}$I. Example protocols have been given wherever possible.

A further section addresses the problem of SPET image display with particular reference to the developments in multi-modality imaging for the brain. This is followed by a discussion of the problems of activity quantification. The limitations of resolution, scatter and attenuation are considered as are the possible solutions to these physical problems.

The final discussion section reviews instrument and radiotracer developments and concludes with a series of recommendations for optimization of brain SPET imaging procedures.

Several important issues are not addressed, not least of which is the problem of consistency in software results from system to system. It is clear that not all systems produce identical or almost identical tomographic reconstructions from the same input data. Such differences must ultimately be removed if an adequate translation of research data into routine clinical practice is to be achieved.

## Single-headed Anger gamma camera systems

Most modern, general purpose Anger gamma camera systems are capable of high-quality brain SPET studies. Former limitations due to gantry and electronic stability have been overcome. Particular emphasis has been placed on allowing imaging in close proximity to the patient using either modifications to the shielding around circular detectors, e.g. the 'cut-away' head, or the use of rectangular fields of view. Further development of collimators to optimize positioning has met with limited success and few single headed gamma cameras can utilize fan beam or cone beam collimator developments. A typical brain acquisition protocol for a single-head gamma camera system is given in Table 1.

*Table 1. Typical brain SPET acquisition protocol*

| | Single head with parallel hole collimators | Triple head with parallel hole collimators | |
|---|---|---|---|
| Collimators | HR | HR | GP |
| No. of views | 64 | 128 | 128 |
| Matrix size | 128 | 64 | 64 |
| Pixel size (mm) | 3.2 | 4.0 | 4.0 |
| Time per view (s) | 30–40 | 20 | 15 |
| Total time (min) | 35–45 | 15 | 11 |
| Counts per view (kcnts)[a] | 50 | 35 | 50 |
| Total counts (kcnts)[a] | 3200 | 4480 | 6400 |

[a] Using 20 per cent energy window with 3 per cent offset, if 600 MBq $^{99m}$Tc-HMPAO were administered.

The limitations of this approach revolve around the problems associated with limited sensitivity. Interventional studies can often only be performed sequentially on static radiotracer distributions with an adequate delay to allow for radiotracer decay. Typically study times of 30–40 min per scan are the maximum that can be tolerated by the patient and the minimum that can be utilized to obtain adequate statistics. Delayed sequential studies therefore require sophisticated techniques for image realignment.

General-purpose gamma cameras have extreme flexibility in detector positioning but this inherent variable geometry leads to one of the major areas of variability on brain SPET imaging. The positioning of the detector often relies heavily on the operator, resulting in wide ranges of radii of rotation for acquisitions. This has a significant effect on the variations in reconstructed resolution and therefore in relative quantification plus visual interpretation from patient to patient and study to study on the same patient. A high-quality procedure is ultimately dependent on the careful positioning of the patient and patient co-operation being achieved over a 30–40 min period. This must be compared with the properties of some of the multiple detector systems described below which offer fixed geometries and sufficient sensitivity to reduce scanning times to 10–15 min with improvements in resolution. Patient positioning times are usually significantly longer with a single gamma camera than with multi-detector and specialized brain SPET systems.

## Multi-detector systems

The realization that any improvements in resolution necessitate a loss in sensitivity has led to the development of SPET systems with more than one gamma camera (commonly three) surrounding the patient's head or body[12,17,28]. The gain factors that can be achieved are dependent on the detector configuration. Table 2 indicates the relative scanning times for possible multi-headed configurations for a 360° set of projections expressed with respect to the time for a single rotating gamma camera.

*Table 2. Relative imaging times for different multi-headed camera configurations expressed with respect to a single gamma camera for 360° acquisition*

| Number of cameras | Relative imaging time |
|---|---|
| 1 Single | 1.0 |
| 2 Opposed | 0.5 |
| 2 Right angles | 0.5 |
| 3 Triangular | 0.33 |
| 4 Square | 0.25 |

It is assumed that camera and collimator characteristics are the same in all cases. Commercial manufacturers offering multi-headed systems are listed in Table 3. The design, configuration and engineering aspects of several multi-detector systems are described below.

### *Medimatic*

The instrument developed by Medimatic[38] uses four banks of 16 crystals arranged in a rectangular array. Here sensitivity has been optimized, through collimator choice, to permit the measurement of cerebral blood flow using dynamic measurements of the washout of $^{133}$Xe. Patients can be studied both supine and erect. This level of sensitivity, although at the price of significant loss of resolution, cannot be achieved by multiple Anger gamma cameras.

*Table 3. Multi-headed/multi-detector SPET systems*

| Company | Model | No. of cameras or detectors | Organ |
|---------|-------|------------------------------|-------|
| ADAC | GENESYS | 2 variable geometry | Brain/body |
| | CERESPECT | Annular crystal | Brain |
| GE | MAXUS | 2 | Brain/body |
| GE | NEUROCAM | 3 | Brain |
| GE | OPTIMA | 2 right angles | Heart |
| HITACHI | SPECT 2000 | 4 | Brain |
| MEDIMATIC | TOMOMATIC | 4 × 16 detectors | Brain |
| PICKER | PRISM | 3 | Brain/body |
| SELO | CERTO96 | 4 | Brain |
| SHIMADZU | SET–031 | 3 rings | Brain |
| SIEMENS | MULTISPECT 2 | 2 | Brain/body |
| SIEMENS | MULTISPECT 3 | 3 | Brain/body |
| SME | 810 | 12 detectors | Brain |
| SOPHA | DST | 2 variable geometry | Brain/body |
| SPRINT | | 1 ring of detectors | Brain |
| TOSHIBA | GCA–9300A | 3 | Brain/body |
| TRIONIX | TRIAD | 3 | Brain/body |

## SME 810

This device was developed in the late 1970s[36]. The gantry assembly contains 12 scanning detectors which are mounted on radial slide rails arranged in a clockwise fashion at 30° intervals around the opening, which has a diameter of 28.5 cm. Each detector consists of a highly focused collimator (focal length 15 cm), a 20 × 13×2.5cm NaI crystal, light guide, photomultiplier tube, amplifier and pulse height analyser. These detectors scan simultaneously, in a rectilinear pattern, to sample a single plane through the brain. The focal point of each detector scans half the region imaged to provide six pairs of data, each sampling the section of interest from six equally spaced angles around the 360°. The system, by concentrating on a single plane, offers considerable gains in sensitivity and speed of scanning such that high resolution imaging of static radiotracers like $^{99m}$Tc-HMPAO and $^{123}$I-IMP can be imaged. The system is capable of imaging energies up to 300 keV, however, with the introduction of increased shielding and high energy collimators, it has also been used to image positron-emitting radiotracers in single photon mode. Full 3-D reconstruction programs have been developed which allow for high resolution reconstructions with significantly decreased cross-talk from adjacent slices due to the improved axial resolution obtained.

## GE Neurocam

The Neurocam system is a brain-dedicated three-headed SPET system which consists of three gamma cameras rigidly fixed in a rotating gantry[25]. The front faces of the cameras form an almost equilateral triangular aperture within which the patient's head is positioned. The size of the aperture is constant; it is large enough to accommodate most adult heads but small enough to ensure close proximity imaging and hence better resolution; the radius of rotation is 123 mm. Each camera has 27 photomultiplier tubes (PMTs) coupled to a 6.5 mm thick NaI(Tl) crystal with adequate shielding for gamma-rays of energy up to 170 keV. The field of view is 200 mm × 176 mm. Unlike single-headed gamma cameras, patient positioning is easily and reproducibly done. The height of the head-rest is fixed with respect to the gantry. The imaging table locks into place when pushed into the aperture. Collimators are light and easily handled. Data acquisition is controlled by an IBM-compatible PC. Data are energy corrected on-line; linearity and uniformity corrections are made off-line for each projection; centre of rotation corrections are made during tomographic reconstruction. Processing is performed on a GE Star computer after data transfer. The Neurocam tomographic sensitivity is about 4× that of the single-headed GE 400XCT camera and its reconstructed resolution is better (Table 6). The Neurocam system is limited to parallel hole collimation due to the small field of view. General purpose, high resolution and ultra high resolution collimators are available. Acquisition can only be performed by 'step and shoot' motion. Rotation is limited to a maximum of 360° giving 3 × 360° data samples. It is only capable of imaging static radiotracer distributions. A 'static radiotracer distribution is here defined as one where the residence half time of the tracer is at least 4–5 times the measurement period.

## *GE Optima*

This system has been primarily designed for optimized cardiac imaging; however, its variable radius of rotation capabilities means that it can readily be adapted for brain SPET applications. It comprises two rectangular detectors 337 × 183 mm using 6.5 mm NaI crystals with 37 photomultiplier tubes. The detectors are arranged at right angles to each other meaning that for 360° SPET applications two complete samples are obtained and averaged post acquisition. It is capable of 'step and shoot' and continuous rotation acquisitions although the speed of rotation would be insufficient for $^{133}$Xe brain blood flow measurements. It is currently supplied with both general purpose and high resolution parallel hole collimators. No fanbeam collimators are available. The advantages of this configuration are that it can be readily adapted for emission/transmission imaging to provide an attenuation map of the brain (see later section on Quantification). The disadvantage of this multi-detector system is that it has a very flexible geometry with regard to radius of rotation and patient positioning relative to the detectors. Careful positioning of patients would be required to minimize variations due to positioning.

## *Toshiba GCA-9300A*

The Toshiba GCA-9300A is a three-headed SPET system for both brain and body tomography[17]. Unlike the Neurocam, the radius of rotation of each camera can be varied independently between 132 and 307 mm. Each camera has 45 PMTs coupled to a 6.5 mm thick NaI(Tl) crystal and is shielded against gamma and X-rays up to 180 keV. The collimators can be changed using custom trolleys. The collimators available at the authors' Institution were the high resolution parallel hole (HR PH) and the super high resolution fanbeam (SHR FB), both cast from lead. The field of view (FOV) is 410 mm × 210 mm (length) with the parallel hole collimators, and 220 mm (diameter) × 210 mm (length) with the fanbeam collimators. The fanbeam collimators have a focal length of 397 mm and must be used with the minimum radius of rotation. Data can be acquired in either 'step and shoot' or 'continuous rotation' mode. In the latter, the cameras are rotated at a constant angular speed, the data being binned into the required number of views. More than one rotation can be performed, the data from each rotation being summed for a given angle; the direction of rotation is reversed between rotations. Data are energy and linearity corrected on-line; uniformity correction of each projection is done prior to tomographic reconstruction. The tomographic sensitivities for the SHR FB and HR PH collimators are almost equal; the fanbeam collimators are used for the brain and the parallel collimators are used for body SPET (Table 7). The SHR FB collimators offer better spatial resolution and marginally better volume sensitivity than the Neurocam HR collimators, demonstrating the advantages of fanbeam geometry.

## *Four-headed Osaka/Hitachi SPECT 2000*

The four-headed Osaka/Hitachi SPECT 2000 is a brain-dedicated instrument[23]. It utilizes four compact gamma cameras rigidly fixed in a square arrangement that can be rotated in either 'step and shoot' or 'continuous rotation' mode. Each camera comprises a NaI(Tl) crystal of thickness 9.0 mm coupled to 30 square PMTs in a $6 \times 5$ array. The distance between the collimator surfaces of opposed detectors is 260 mm, hence 130 mm radius of rotation (compared to 123 mm for the Neurocam and 132 mm for the GCA-9300A); the field of view is $220 \times 170$ mm, similar to that of the Neurocam. With HR collimators, the reconstructed spatial resolution of the Osaka system at the centre of the FOV in air is 7.0 mm Full Width at Half Maximum of the line spread function (FWHM) compared to 9.0 mm for the Neurocam. However, with the GP collimators, the Osaka reconstructed resolution at the centre is 13.0 mm compared to 10.7 mm for the Neurocam. Because of their higher sensitivity (hence poorer spatial resolution) these collimators should more appropriately be called high sensitivity (HS) and be used only for dynamic brain SPET. Here a dynamic tracer distribution measurement needs to be made at intervals of a fifth to a tenth of the biological half-life of the radiotracer.

## CERESPECT

The annular single-crystal brain camera (CERESPECT) consists of a stationary annular NaI(Tl) crystal and a rotating collimator system[11,36]. The FOV is 217 mm diam. $\times$ 106 mm in the axial direction. The internal diameter of the crystal is 310 mm and its thickness 8 mm. It is viewed by 63 PMTs arranged in three rings. Each PMT output is digitized so that all subsequent processing is digitally performed (including position computation, linearity and energy corrections). The concentric collimator system comprises three parallel hole collimators viewing the head from three angles simultaneously. The reconstructed spatial resolution, for the general purpose high resolution collimator, is 7.5 mm at the centre in air and the tomographic volume sensitivity is 27.0 kcps/MBq/ml/cm. The system is shielded to 275 keV. This system is capable of imaging static and time varying tracer distributions including $^{133}$Xe. Again such system optimization permits studies of the patient in erect and supine positions.

## Trionix TRIAD

The Trionix TRIAD system comprises three rectangular detectors arranged as a triangle on an open ring type gantry[28]. The detectors can be moved radially to permit both high resolution brain and body studies, the radius of rotation varying between 125 mm and 280 mm. Each detector utilizes 49, 60 mm hexagonal PMTs to give a useful field of view with parallel hole collimation of 400 mm $\times$ 220 mm. A 9.5 mm NaI crystal is used along with adequate shielding to provide imaging over the range 50–400 keV. Digital corrections are provided for energy, linearity and flood field distortions together with corrections for relative X-Y detector shifts. A range of fanbeam collimators are available to provide a tomographic field of view of 250 mm $\times$ 220 mm (axial) for brain imaging with system resolutions between 5.7 mm and 9.5 mm 10 cm from the collimator surface. Low energy collimators are rated to 160 keV. The gantry is capable of continuous or 'step and shoot' acquisition with rotation through a maximum of 380°. A full 360° acquisition can be obtained in 5 s. An automatic patient contouring feature has recently been introduced on this system which dynamically adjusts the detector to patient distance during acquisition.

## Picker PRISM

As for the Triad, the Prism system comprises three rectangular detectors each with 49 PMTs and a 9 mm thick NaI(Tl) scintillation crystal. The useful planar field of view of each detector is 400 mm $\times$ 240 mm (axial). These are arranged in a triangular configuration with radial motion allowed to provide for both brain and body imaging. This provides an open ring configuration rather than a tunnel gantry. A range of parallel collimation is available for imaging to 400 keV. Fanbeam collimators are available for high-resolution brain imaging with the field of view being reduced to 300 mm $\times$ 240 mm. No collimators are available for dynamic tracer measurements using $^{133}$Xe. The distance from the edge of the useful field of the UFOV to the edge of the detector housing has been reduced to 6.5 cm to enable easier patient positioning for brain imaging.

### *Siemens Multispect3*

This system has three large field of view detectors with collimation and shielding to allow acquisitions up to 400 keV. The detectors (FOV 31 × 41 cm are arranged as a variable aperture triangle within a double ring style gantry. It uses a 9.5 mm crystal with 76, 50 mm diameter photomultiplier tubes per detector. It has a minimum sampling time of 15 s for 360° rotation. This system also uses a series of infra-red beams and detectors to aid the set-up of patient body contouring. Such a system of infra-red beams could also be used to provide patient/couch outlines for attenuation correction purposes during reconstruction.

From an analysis of the above systems it is clear that the gain in sensitivity achieved by using more than one camera simultaneously has given additional flexibility to collimator designers in reaching a compromise between sensitivity and resolution. These developments will continue with the introduction of new collimator configurations aimed at further exploitation of sensitivity in relation to improved resolution. Further developments will also reflect the need to introduce measured attenuation and scatter correction methods in SPET reconstruction.

## Performance characteristics of brain SPET systems

The optimization of data from brain SPET studies is dependent on the physical characteristics of the system, upon applications of the technology and the clinical problem. The limitations imposed by the system can be readily understood through the analysis of key components of the imaging process. However, the optimum utilization of the system capabilities is dependent on the user correctly defining/specifying the acquisition, analysis and display protocols. Here the definition of a 'correct' protocol is more difficult and open to significant variation in the available literature.

In this section those parameters defined by the system which significantly influence the SPET imaging process have been analysed. These parameters include spatial and energy resolution and also temporal resolution. The latter usually relates to the count rate performance of the detector but in this context also relates to the minimum data acquisition period for a complete 3-D dataset. Related to spatial resolution is the absolute 3-D sensitivity of the detector. Depending on the system configuration the radius of rotation of the detectors may be fixed or variable. Those systems with a fixed radius of rotation often enable this parameter to be optimized. Other parameters which may influence the choice of instrument are field of view and energy range.

### *Spatial resolution*

The tomographic spatial resolution of a SPET system as measured in air is primarily determined by the system planar resolution. For some systems there may be significant degradation of planar resolution in the tomographic process. It is generally accepted that the tomographic resolution of a system at the centre of the tomographic field of view should not be greater than 1.1 times the planar resolution at an equal distance. The resolution at the centre of the tomographic field of view is clearly highly dependent on the radius of rotation of the detectors. For brain studies it is therefore essential for the radius of rotation to be minimized and this requires adequate operator training to optimize the acquisition process. There is normally significant variation of resolution between the centre and the edge of the field of view due to the variation of resolution with distance from the collimator. This leads to a non-uniform sampling of the tomographic volume which in turn leads to errors in accurate quantification. The figures presented to the following section are based on the resolution at the centre of the field of view and therefore represent the worst resolution within a tomographic slice. For most area detectors this is equivalent to the spatial resolution in the axial direction, however, for the single slice, multi-detector systems, the axial resolution may vary markedly from the in-plane resolution leading to a non-isotropic sampling of the 3-D volume.

### Tomographic sensitivity

Tomographic volume sensitivity is variously defined within the literature. Any measurement is dependent upon the object imaged, its radius and length relative to the detector field of view, the energy window used and the energy resolution of the detection system. The measurement further requires the method for the determination of data acquisition time to be closely defined. The measurements presented below are for a 20 cm diameter cylinder of length 25 cm. The figures are the maximum values which could be obtained and do not take account of losses due to detector motion and initialization. For some systems these losses may be highly significant. The losses cannot be expressed as a fixed percentage since it will be dependent on the imaging time per projection. It is clear that systems capable of acquiring whilst the detector is in constant motion allow this parameter to be optimized.

### Resolution vs sensitivity

SPET systems have a characteristic resolution volume, determined by the in-plane and axial resolutions. This volume is approximately cylindrical, of height $2 \times$ FWHM (axial) and diameter $2 \times$ FWHM (in-plane). Reconstructed images of these objects will reflect both the size and radioactive concentration of the object. However, for objects smaller than this the signal is blurred so as to occupy the entire resolution volume. This is known as the partial volume effect. The total counts in the source will still be conserved, even though the activity per pixel (voxel) is decreased. It is a resolution rather than a sensitivity problem. This effect can be compensated for if the size of the object can be measured independently allowing a recovery coefficient to be applied. This problem is particularly severe in the brain where grey and white matter are so convolved at a scale below the resolving power of the methodology that accurate determination of radioactive concentrations in each tissue type independently is impossible. Average values are always obtained. The need to maximize the resolving power of the detector as well as its sensitivity in order to minimize the partial volume effect is clear. This will lead directly to an increased ability to quantify absolutely activity per unit volume in structures of dimensions typically found in the brain.

The utilization of a system's performance characteristics (principally governed by the collimation used) will depend on the maximum permissible administered dose allowed, the maximum practical scanning time and the clinical problem to be investigated. The influence of the clinical problem is important since it will define the signal-to-noise ratio required in the resultant reconstructions to obtain statistically significant results. This may not relate to the absolute quantification of activity concentrations per image pixel but rather to relative count rates within relatively large regions of interest. The signal-to-noise ratio of interest is therefore that within a region often considerably larger than a unit voxel.

Resolution and sensitivity could effectively be replaced by the terms signal and noise. As described above, the finite resolution of the system may result in significant errors in the measured activity or signal. The limitations imposed by the system sensitivity, patient dose and scan duration will result in statistical errors in the reconstructed data or noise. The ratio of these two components in the reconstructed image can be used as a measure of image quality for a particular clinical problem.

The interaction of these two system characteristics and the impact on system design can be seen by reference to data obtained from both single and triple-headed Anger gamma camera systems.

*Table 4. Comparison of collimator parameters for the GE 400XCT single rotating gamma camera, the GE Neurocam brain-dedicated three-headed system, the CERESPECT brain-dedicated annular single crystal camera, the Picker Prism head and body three-headed system, and Siemens Multispect3*

|  |  | Hole size (mm) | Septal thickness (mm) | Hole length (mm) |
|---|---|---|---|---|
| GE 400 XCT | GP | 2.5 | 0.3 | 41 |
|  | HR | 1.8 | 0.3 | 40 |
| Neurocam | GP | 1.8 | 0.2 | 31.5 |
|  | HR | 1.4 | 0.2 | 31.5 |
|  | UHR | 1.4 | 0.2 | 38.5 |
| CERESPECT | HR | 1.0 | 0.18 | 24.0 |
| Picker PRISM | GP | 1.6 | 0.24 | 25.4 |
|  | HR | 1.4 | 0.18 | 27.0 |
|  | UHR | 1.4 | 0.15 | 34.9 |
| Multispect3 | HR | 1.13 | 0.16 | 23.6 |
|  | UHR | 1.16 | 0.13 | 35.6 |

Table 4 compares the manufacturer's construction specifications of collimators for the GE 400XCT single rotating camera, the three-headed GE Neurocam, the CERESPECT system and the Picker Prism head and body three-headed system. Table 5 compares the measured planar sensitivity and planar resolution for the GE 400XCT, GE Neurocam and GCA-9300A. Table 6 compares the tomographic resolution and volume sensitivity for the three systems. The planar sensitivity and resolution of Table 5 are directly dependent on the data provided in Table 4. Similarly, the tomographic performance figures of Table 6 are a direct consequence of the planar characteristics of Table 5.

*Table 5. Comparison of measured planar point source sensitivity and spatial resolution for the GE 400XCT camera, the GE Neurocam and the Toshiba GCA-9300A*

|  |  | Planar sensitivity (cps/MBq) | Planar resolution FWHM (mm) |
|---|---|---|---|
| GE 400XCT | GP | 142 | 10.4 |
|  | HR | 82 | 8.3 |
| Neurocam | GP | $130 \times 3$ | 9.6 |
|  | HR | $75 \times 3$ | 7.9 |
| GCA-9300A | HR | $75 \times 3$ | 8.0 |

Table 6. *Comparison of tomographic performance of GE 400XCT, GE Neurocam and Toshiba GCA-9300A for* $^{99m}Tc$ *using 20 per cent symmetric energy window*

| | | Collimator | | |
| --- | --- | --- | --- | --- |
| | | GE 400XCT | GE Neurocam | Toshiba |
| Tomographic volume sensitivity (kcps/MBq/ml/cm) | GP | 12.8 | 50.7 | |
| | HR | 7.6 | 30.0 | 33.8 |
| | SHR FB | | | 34.8 |
| Tomographic spatial resolution in air (FWHM mm)* | GP | 11.7 | 10.7 | |
| | HR | 10.3 | 9.0 | 10.2 |
| | SHR FB | 7.8 | | 7.6 |

*Radius of rotation: GE 400XCT 130mm, GE Neurocam 123 mm, GCA-9300A 132 mm.

### Temporal resolution

Temporal resolution in this context is defined as the minimum time taken to obtain a complete 360° sample of an activity distribution. The tomographic process requires that the radiotracer distribution does not change throughout the acquisition process. Changes may be caused by patient motion or tracer kinetics within the brain. The potential to obtain rapid 360° samples will assist in both these areas. The development of radiotracers for the brain has been focused by the need to obtain a functional marker which has a fixed distribution for a time sufficient to enable imaging to be accomplished in one pass with a single Anger gamma camera. This design constraint has led to a series of markers with which it is difficult to perform rapid sequential intervention studies due to the long retention time within the brain. Such studies could be performed with a tracer of short residence time within the organ if a high-sensitivity detector capable of rapid 360° sampling was available. Such detectors have been produced using purpose built detectors and applied particularly to the measurement of blood flow using $^{133}$Xe. It is now possible to provide similar characteristics with $^{99m}$Tc compounds which would require complete 360° samples to be taken in 5–10 s.

Where patient motion is a potential problem the acquisition of multiple, rapid 360° samples may provide useful data prior to patient motion, whereas the use of a single, slow acquisition is useless if the patient moves when even 90 per cent of the study is complete. Rapid, sequential, CW/CCW 360° samples also alleviate the problem of changing radioactive distributions where an average 'static' image is required.

### Energy resolution

The importance of the energy resolution of a detector is often overlooked. As a result the improvements in this parameter on a number of modern systems are often not exploited. The range of values of this parameter for current gamma camera detectors is approximately 9.5–12.5 per cent for $^{99m}$Tc.

Typically, the poorer energy resolution systems have been operated with wide (20 per cent) pulse height analyser windows. This action has been taken to maintain count rates since using smaller or offset windows results in significant decreases in apparent sensitivity and often introduces significant non-uniformity in the response of the detector to a plane source. However, the use of a 20 per cent pulse height window on a system with an energy resolution of 9.5 per cent, when used in clinical practice will result in the inclusion of increased levels of scattered photons causing significant decreases in reconstructed image contrast. Systems with good energy resolution should be used with reduced (15–17.5 per cent) pulse height analyser windows and may even be operated with offset windows. For the GE Neurocam system the change from a symmetric window (112–168 keV) to an offset window (117–172 keV) resulted in a 25 per cent change in measured grey to white matter ratios in the Hoffman 3-D brain phantom. It is essential that the uniformity response of the detector is checked under these operating conditions. Where uniformity calibrations are used in the tomographic imaging process these must be derived from images taken under the same operating conditions.

### Energy range

With few exceptions the energy range of Anger gamma camera-based tomographic devices has been restricted to energies below 200 keV and may even be lower, optimized for $^{99m}$Tc. This may be perceived as an unnecessary compromise since it precludes the use of radionuclides such as $^{111}$In and $^{68}$Ga and $^{131}$I. The increased sensitivity of the multi-detector devices will certainly permit the imaging of radiotracers with low accumulation in the brain of which $^{201}$Tl-, $^{68}$Ga- and iodine-labelled compounds are examples. $^{201}$Tl presents particular difficulties since its low energy emissions are difficult to detect accurately and system performance is often degraded at these energies.

### Detector field of view

The useful field of view (UFOV) of the detector is related to the overall sensitivity of the device in clinical imaging. The greater the area of detector which can be exposed to the activity distribution within the patient, the greater the tomographic sensitivity of the system. The design choice appears to be between small detectors arranged close to the brain using parallel hole collimators and the use of larger detectors positioned at a greater distance from the patient but capable of using either parallel hole, fan beam and eventually cone beam collimators. The gains in sensitivity which can be achieved using parallel hole collimators are simply in proportion to the number of detectors for 360° acquisitions. The use of fan beam and cone beam collimators enable more crystal to be exposed and hence the gain in sensitivity now becomes a function of the detector size. For fan beam collimators the width of the detector in the transaxial plane is the determinant factor, for cone beam collimators it is the overall area of the detector. Typical gains which might be achieved are shown in Table 7.

*Table 7. Relative sensitivities for different collimator designs. Sensitivities are expressed relative to a parallel hole collimator. It is assumed that each would provide the same spatial resolution*

| Collimator | Relative sensitivity |
|---|---|
| Parallel | 1.0 |
| Fan beam | 1.4 – 1.6 |
| Cone beam | 2.0 –2.5 |

### Contrast

Contrast is variously defined within the literature. It is a measure of the accuracy of activity concentration measurements when compared to the true values. A reduction in contrast will also impinge upon relative activity measurements as well as difference measurements producing a systematic error. The reproducibility of a measurement will primarily be affected by the random errors associated with the technique. Contrast is a measure which is dependent on the entire set of system and user variables. It encompasses effects due to spatial resolution, energy resolution, pulse height analyser settings, acquisition and processing protocols, system calibration as well as attenuation and scatter within the object imaged. Without a knowledge of the original distribution a measure of accuracy of reconstruction cannot be and is not normally made.

Contrast is usually used in a comparative way to compare the response of a system to a known object under various operating conditions. Generally contrast (C) is defined for two regions within an object as:

$$C = (R_1 - R_2)/(R_1 + R_2)$$

Where $R_1$ and $R_2$ represent the average counts/pixel in each of two regions usually adjacent to each other or one encompasses the other, e.g. target and background. For two line sources with equal activity concentrations contrast has been defined as follows:

$$C = (Peak\ Cnts - Valley\ Cnts)/(Peak\ Cnts + Valley\ Cnts)$$

The effect of system and user defined parameters on the contrast within the reconstructed image is often overlooked and underestimated. This can most easily be illustrated from results obtained with simulations of the Hoffman 3-D brain phantom[18] where grey to white matter ratios are fixed by the construction of the phantom. Using simulations based on this anthropomorphic test object Kim *et al.*[21] demonstrated that without attenuation, scatter or noise a circumferential profile around the cortex of the brain yielded values varying by factors of 2.5–3.0 from a uniform activity distribution but with differing volumes of distribution. These simulations were based on the resolution characteristics of two different SPET systems, a Trionix Triad with ultra-high resolution parallel hole collimators and a Strichman 810 multi-detector scanner. The results of the simulations for the grey to white matter ratios were of the order of 2.5:1 rather than the 5:1 of the phantom. These simulations were confirmed by physical measurements using the phantom and the two SPET systems.

The above results are further supported by measurements made on a Toshiba GCA-9300A

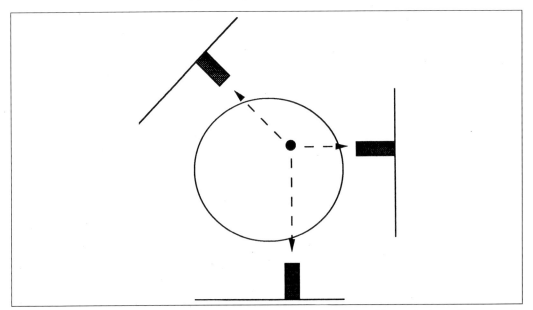

*Fig. 1. Demonstration of the principles of tomographic data acquisition. Theoretical one dimensional (1-D) projections acquired by a position sensitive detector rotating around an object comprising a point source of radioactivity.*

triple-headed system using a Hoffman 3-D phantom with expected grey/white matter ratios of 4:1. The data presented below are all from high count acquisitions for a number of different acquisition and/or processing conditions. The data is obtained from the same transaxial slice through the thalami and basal ganglia. The average grey/white matter ratios obtained using square regions of interest (ROIs), in the same positions, for each different set of conditions varied between 1.98:1 and 2.43:1. The size of the ROI was 8.7 mm × 8.7 mm², corresponding to about 1 × the FWHM spatial resolution. All values are significantly less than 4:1 due to the partial volume effect. There was no quantitative difference in grey/white matter ratio between step or continuous acquisition modes, for either parallel or fanbeam collimators. Adding projection data from more than one rotation causes a reduction in grey/white matter ratio. In the presence of high counts (and hence low noise), a higher cut-off frequency filter yields a higher grey/white matter ratio; even so the maximum value obtained using a symmetric window was only about 2.3 with a Butterworth filter, power 8, 0.8 cycles/cm cut-off frequency. Use of an asymmetric energy window (3 per cent offset) gave no improvement for the parallel hole collimators and only a 5.6 per cent improvement for fanbeam collimators (2.32:1 and 2.43:1). There was a slight visual improvement in image quality with the asymmetric window using the SHR FB collimators.

In routine clinical brain studies using the SHR FB collimators, the total counts acquired are typically about 4–5 Mcnts and the average grey/white matter ratio is only about 1.7 (using the Butterworth prefilter with power 8 with 0.6 cycles/cm critical frequency and no attenuation correction). A similar value (1.73) was obtained with a 4.0 Mcnts acquisition using the Hoffman 3-D brain phantom.

The influence of the reconstruction software must not be overlooked. Recent results obtained by the authors suggest that significant differences in activity ratios are obtained for the same input data and equivalent filters on different computer systems. Further standardization work will be required in this area if reproducible results are to be obtained between centres.

**Acquisition and processing protocols**

Whilst the performance characteristics considered above were treated as separate components of the tomographic process it is in combination that they determine the final image. It is in the acquisition and processing protocol that the clinical problem is of importance since the size of the region to be quantified will define the level of resolution required in the reconstructed data. For the brain almost all studies seek to address changes in structures which are well below achievable resolutions and thus collimation, spatial sampling and filters must be chosen so as to retain as much resolution as possible within the final image.

The principles of tomographic data acquisition and image reconstruction are illustrated in Figs. 1 and 2 respectively. For a point source of radioactivity, three one-dimensional (1-D) projections are shown in Fig. 1 as would have been obtained by a 1-D array of discrete, well-collimated detectors viewing the 'object' in the directions indicated. With a parallel hole collimator, each measurement in a given pixel can be considered to represent the sum of radioactivity along the 'lines' through the patient that correspond to the collimator holes of that pixel. A given row of pixels in each of the projections corresponds to the slice perpendicular to the camera and axis of rotation; this slice is said to be sampled by this set of measurements. The above description is true in the absence of attenuation and scatter and assumes an ideal detector exhibiting perfect spatial resolution – conditions that do not apply in practice. Nevertheless, it sets the foundation of SPET data acquisition, namely that data must be acquired along well defined 'lines'. It also sets the foundation of SPET reconstruction because accurate knowledge is required of these lines and directions along which the data were acquired. Mathematically, an exact reconstruction can

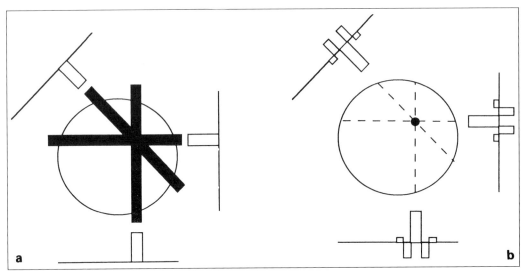

*Fig. 2. Demonstration of the principles of tomographic reconstruction using the filtered backprojection method. (a) Using the projection data of Fig. 1, backprojection leads to the visualization of the point source by superimposition. A star-like artefact is generated. (b) Filtering modifies the projection data so that after backprojection, the artefact is no longer evident.*

only be achieved provided that the slice to be reconstructed is sampled (i.e. measurements taken) along an infinite number of lines and directions. In practice, measurements are taken along finite lines and finite directions. How effective the sampling is determines image quality. Hence the sampling pattern implemented by the design of a given system is critical.

There are two basic methods for reconstruction:

(a) filtered back projection;

(b) iterative reconstruction.

Filtered back projection is an analytical technique which, under ideal circumstances, should produce an exact solution. The process is illustrated in Fig. 2 and can be divided into two parts, the first of which is back-projection, which can be seen as the inverse of the acquisition process. The pixel data, representing the sum along a line from a particular direction through the object, is reprojected onto the reconstruction image plane along the same direction. The data are reprojected as if the original data were uniformly distributed since this is the most reasonable assumption given that the distribution is unknown. When this process is repeated for all angles a superposition of data is obtained which leads to a blurred image of the original object where each point is represented by a star pattern. This blurring can be removed by the second stage of the reconstruction process, that of filtering. This again has two components: the first is a filter which specifically removes the blurring, the second is a filter which reduces errors due to inconsistencies in the data particularly those due to statistical counting errors. These two steps are often applied independently and the user is given control over the level of filtering applied to reduce statistical noise in the final image. These are referred to in more detail in the sub-section on reconstruction.

*Acquisition*

Whether in planar imaging or in SPET, the pixel size defines the spatial sampling. Optimally, it should be < FWHM (mm)/3, e.g. about 3–4 mm for a SPET system that is characterized by a 10 mm FWHM resolution for a given imaging task. The angular sampling interval is defined by the number of projections in 360°. In order to ensure similar spatial and angular sampling at the circumference of the reconstruction region, the angular interval should be such that the arc length is equal to the spatial sampling interval. In the brain, this would ensure optimal sampling of the outer cortex, and with a 4 mm spatial sampling interval, the angular sampling interval should be about 3°. It is clear that with the introduction of higher resolution collimators the spatial and angular sampling should be increased using these guidelines to prevent degradation of the data at the acquisition stage.

At the authors' Institution the HR parallel hole collimators are used for most studies on the Neurocam and the SHR fanbeam collimators have been used for all brain studies on the GCA-9300A. The most common data acquisition parameters on the Neurocam are: 128 projections, 64 × 64 (pixel size 4.0 mm), 20–40 s per projection. Since at each step during the rotation, three projections are acquired simultaneously, the total acquisition time for a typical $^{99m}$Tc-HMPAO study with 20 s per projection takes about 15 min. The most common data acquisition parameters on the GCA-9300A are: 90 fanbeam 256 × 256 projections converted to 60 parallel 128 × 128 projections (pixel size 1.735 mm), 30–60 s per projection. Acquisition protocols and resulting counts and acquisition times are compared for the GE 400XCT gamma camera, Neurocam, GCA-9300A and SME 810 in Table 8.

### Reconstruction

Most systems reconstruct the images using a filtered backprojection method as described above. The backprojection method introduces a blurring of the image and, for perfect data, this can be corrected by filtering with the inverse of the blurring function. For systems which use a Fourier method for reconstruction this equates to a Ramp filter in frequency space. The disadvantage of this filter is that it enhances high spatial frequency noise in the image. It is thus necessary to apply a second filter which will suppress these high frequency components whilst retaining sufficient information in the reconstructed image.

These latter filters are usually of two types: firstly, low pass filters which only smooth the data, such as the Hanning and Butterworth filters. Secondly, those which seek to provide some enhancement of low frequencies whilst still retaining the smoothing function at high frequencies. These include the Metz and Weiner filters. All the filters require the specification of one or more parameters to define the degree of smoothing by defining the shape of the filter.

*Table 8. Comparison of acquisition protocols for $^{99m}$Tc-HMPAO brain perfusion studies using the GE 400XCT camera, GE Neurocam, Toshiba GCA-9300A and SME810*

|  | GE 400XCT | GE Neurocam | GE Neurocam | Toshiba GCA 9300A | SME |
|---|---|---|---|---|---|
| Collimators | HR | HR | GP | SHR FB | HR |
| No. of views | 64 | 128 | 128 | 90→60 | 12 |
| Energy window, offset % | 20.3 | 20.3 | 20.3 | 20.0 | 115–170 keV |
| Matrix size | 128 | 64 | 64 | 256→128 | 128 |
| Pixel size (mm) | 3.2 | 4.0 | 4.0 | 1.735 | 1.6 |
| Time per view (s) | 30–40 | 20 | 15 | 30 | 150 per slice |
| Total time (min) | 35–45 | 15 | 11 | 15 | 50 for 20 slices |
| Counts per view (kcnts) | 50 | 35 | 50 | 55 | 1500 per slice |
| Total counts (Mcnts) | 3.2 | 4.5 | 6.4 | 5.1 | 30 for 20 slices |

These filters can be applied to each reconstructed slice independently or in 2-D to the projection data prior to reconstruction. This latter approach is recommended since it results in a more homogeneous noise spectrum throughout the reconstructed volume. It also takes into account the correlation that exists between adjacent slices. The reconstruction should be performed on single pixel width data, especially where the reconstructed volume is to be reorientated to provide sections of standard projections through the brain. Once the reorientation has been performed the section data can be combined for increased statistical accuracy and display. If an image magnification step is required it is best that this step be performed during the backprojection process. This obviates the need for a second interpolation step post reconstruction.

Within the reconstruction process compensation must be made for scatter and attenuation. For most systems compensation for scatter and attenuation is combined. In theory this is not an appropriate action but is sufficient if absolute quantification of activity is not required. The process involves the delineation of the edge of the body using either a manual or automatic technique, usually based on the edge of the radioactive distribution. This is taken to coincide with the edge of the scattering volume of the body. For the brain, within this region a uniform attenuation is assumed. The value used is reduced from that required to compensate for attenuation alone since the inclusion of scattered photons reduces the apparent attenuation. Typically a value of 0.12 cm$^{-1}$ is used for the linear attenuation coefficient. If a scatter correction technique is applied prior to attenuation correction then a value nearer 0.15 cm$^{-1}$ must be used. Further discussion of methods for scatter and attenuation correction are discussed in the section headed Quantification.

Typically, at the authors' Institute, tomographic reconstruction of $^{99m}$Tc-HMPAO brain perfusion studies is performed using the filtered backprojection method. Projection data acquired on the GE 400XCT are prefiltered using the Hanning filter with cut-off frequency 0.8 cycles/cm and backprojection is done using the ramp filter. On the Neurocam, the cut-off frequency is in the range 1.0–1.2 cycles/cm because of the higher counts acquired; alternatively, the Butterworth prefilter may be used; attenuation correction assumes a uniform linear attenuation coefficient of 0.12 cm$^{-1}$. On the GCA-9300A, the Butterworth prefilter is used and backprojection is done using the ramp filter; no attenuation correction is performed with the fanbeam collimators. For both systems, horizontal slices parallel to the OM-line as well as sagittal and coronal slices are generated from the transaxial dataset, although the process is not limited to orthogonal planes. On the SME 810, a single slice at a time is scanned with the gantry inclined so that the slice is parallel to the OM-line, multiple parallel slices are acquired sequentially. Provided that the slice to slice spacing is of the same order as the pixel size, the slice data can be reorientated to provide sections at any angle through the 3-D dataset. Reconstruction is a two-part process: an initial analytical reconstruction followed by an iterative convolution step.

## Display

The tomographic process results in a large number of images which have to be adequately displayed and reviewed. Brain SPET is no exception. A systematic display protocol is essential to achieve reproducible interpretation of data. This is taken to include the realignment of data to standard planes for comparison with control subjects. This normally involves the display of three orthogonal planes although it should not be restricted to this mode. The use and definition of colour scale and upper and lower count display levels also need careful consideration. It is thought inappropriate to subtract background due to the artificially enhanced contrast in SPET images.

The functional maps obtained from SPET images of the brain are of lower spatial resolution than the anatomical maps of CT or MRI. Anatomical information can only be inferred from SPET images. A valid anatomical map can aid in the interpretation of the functional map. For example, areas of cortex which are reduced in volume will lead to decreases in radiotracer signal due to the increased dilution caused by the partial volume effect. By comparing the results from an anatomical measurement and a functional measurement a more accurate interpretation of the functional map may be achieved. There is now considerable interest in combining these anatomical and functional maps using computer processing. Three major applications have been identified[31]. Firstly, the improvement in the interpretation of functional maps through better anatomical localization[15,16]. Secondly, the use of the anatomical maps to better identify regions or volumes of interest for the interpretation and quantification of functional maps[6,7]. Thirdly, to combine the information to produce a new representation of the data. CT data can be used to correct the functional maps for attenuation effects[9]. CT and MRI maps can also be used to assist in the recovery of resolution in the functional maps. The reduction in the partial volume effect by deconvolution of the functional map by an anatomical map has been reported by a number of workers[22].

Techniques for accurate alignment of images are being developed. The aim is to avoid the use of surface markers in each modality as an aid to realignment but rather to use the data itself. It is clear that these techniques will develop rapidly with the increase in computer processing and display speeds and the introduction of data networks.

## Quantification

The quantification of radioactive concentrations is dependent on and limited by a number of factors. These include Poisson noise, scatter, attenuation, a finite non-stationary detector response (variable resolution within the imaged volume) and sampling limitations as well as reconstruction filter characteristics. As mentioned earlier, for absolute measurements accurate scatter and attenuation corrections are required. In relation to the improvements that can be obtained by the use of high resolution collimators the limits imposed by a finite resolution have a large influence on the measurement of activity concentrations within the brain as discussed in the sub-section on contrast.

The tomographic process assumes a stationary distribution of radiotracer during the acquisition period. Variations in radioactive distributions during the period of the measurement will degrade the measurement. Radioactive decay can be corrected for by a simple multiplicative correction, however, the variations due to changes in signal-to-noise ratio caused by different numbers of photons detected will remain. This limitation can be removed if multiple fast SPET acquisitions are performed and summed prior to reconstruction to provide a mean projection image set. Such facilities are available on a number of brain SPET systems.

Quantification is considered below under three headings. Firstly, the measurement of size and volume of features within the radioactive distribution. Secondly, the measurement of relative activity concentrations between regions of the brain. Thirdly, the measurement of absolute tracer concentration in units of MBq/ml.

### Size and volume

The measurement of the linear size and volume of distribution of a radiotracer or an abnormality in a distribution is primarily limited by the finite resolution of the detector and the statistical errors in the reconstruction as discussed in the section headed 'Performance characteristics of brain SPET systems' earlier. The accuracy with which volumes of interest can be defined will be dependent on the accuracy with which edge detection algorithms can be applied and hence on the signal-to-noise ratio in the image and the contrast range within the image. This latter measure is also a function of attenuation and scatter. The partial volume effect defined by the finite resolution of the imaging process will require different threshold algorithms to be applied for different size structures. The factors which influence size and volume calculations are thus a combination of system and user defined parameters. The spatial resolution is the major system parameter whereas the user can significantly affect the result in the choice of reconstruction filter, dimension of the filter (1-D, 2-D or 3-D) and acquisition pixel size and reconstructed voxel size. These parameters have been investigated by King et al.[24] and Lee et al.[27]. They conclude that resolution and sample size have greatest influence on volume and size measurements. Since resolution is primarily governed by collimator choice these findings raise the question of how far sensitivity can be sacrificed in relation to gains in resolution. This problem has been addressed by Muehllehner[33] and more recently Fahey et al.[8] These investigators sought to identify the relationship between resolution, sensitivity and SPET image quality. The definition of image quality is not easy. Muehllehner used the human observer to identify the 'best' image whereas, in addition, Fahey used a statistical method based on the normalized mean square error (NMSE). The conclusion of both investigators was that image quality could be improved by the use of higher resolution collimators at the expense of significant loss in sensitivity. Madsen et al.[30] indicated that the NMSE was a good indicator of image preference and that there was an optimum choice of collimator based on resolution and total counts within the image. For $^{123}$I studies the optimal spatial resolution, derived in this manner, was found to be about 8–9 mm whereas for $^{99m}$Tc-based studies, the optimal resolution was predicted to be 6–7 mm. They indicate that improvements in sensitivity with dedicated devices could lead to resolutions of 4–5 mm FWHM. In general for brain imaging the highest possible resolution collimator available should be used. Several clinical studies have been reported using ultra-high resolution collimators yielding systems resolutions of 6.5–7.5 mm FWHM.

*Relative activity concentrations*

This approach has been utilized widely in relation to brain SPET since it is less sensitive to the limitations imposed by the physical problems of scatter and attenuation of the *in vivo* radioactive distribution. Typical measures include the comparison of counts from the left and right hemispheres of the brain, either on a slice by slice basis, or from the total brain volume. A comparison of counts from regions of interest, either regular or irregular to a reference anatomical area such as the cerebellum or visual cortex, have also been used. Ranges obtained from a group of normal subjects, preferably age matched, are used to provide comparative data for patient investigations. Such techniques are dependent on many factors. They include, amongst others, the question of control subjects for different disease groups, the adequate definition of anatomical regions for region of interest placement, the size of the region, the identification of the reference site and its freedom from other disease process. Many of these can be overcome within a single centre with care and operator training. However, the comparison of results with other centres and the use of control data from other centres is a major problem which is not readily overcome. For centres using identical equipment for acquisition and processing, including identical reconstruction filter specifications then transfer of data should possible. For centres using different detector systems with different system resolutions, different acquisition protocols and in particular acquisition radius of rotation, different reconstruction software and filters, these will almost certainly lead to different results with more or less discrimination of disease states being the result.

For the results from such techniques to become widely used and distributed there must be rapid progress to the standardization of acquisition and processing techniques. In the first instance groups using equivalent equipment should collaborate to provide control subjects for comparison purposes. The standardization of reconstruction software will require the definitions of standards against which to test the results of particular filter functions.

### Absolute activity concentrations

The measurement of absolute tracer concentrations remains the elusive goal of nuclear medicine and SPET in particular. The important and difficult problems of attenuation and scatter must be addressed if absolute activities are to be measured. From a single measurement of the emitted photons from an organ it will not be possible to obtain a unique solution to the absolute activity distribution. A second independent measurement of attenuation will be required to deduce the emission and attenuation maps correctly. The correction for attenuation without correction for the scattered photons will be insufficient for accurate quantification. If these two corrections can be adequately performed the problems posed by the finite resolution of the process remain and will impose limits equivalent to those referred to above under size and volume quantification.

### Attenuation correction

Several techniques have been proposed for the correction of photon attenuation and include pre-processing of the projection data, modification of the back projection process, post-reconstruction correction techniques and modified iterative reconstruction techniques. These have recently been reviewed by Blokland *et al.*[3]

As discussed earlier, without an independent measurement of attenuation the majority of reconstructions use a single modified linear attenuation coefficient applied within an organ edge defined by the radioactive distribution or the scatter distribution. An intermediate step between a uniform attenuation coefficient and the direct measurement of an attenuation map is to use an attenuation map taken from an atlas of CT scans using sex and size matching for particular anatomical regions. These techniques have been successfully applied by Fleming[9].

An accurate reconstruction requires a measurement of the attenuation distribution within the patient. Much of the earlier work was based on the measurement of the transmission map prior to injecting the patient with a radiotracer. An intrinsic measurement using a point source and fanbeam geometry has been proposed. The use of a uniform radioactive flood source both with and without collimation at the source and with a parallel hole collimator on the camera have been used[2,10]. It was concluded that it was necessary firstly to have a measurement of the narrow beam attenuation coefficients, and secondly to collimate both source and detector to exclude the effects of scatter during transmission. The technique was developed to use a highly collimated scanning line source[39] to provide a lower dose to the patient and staff and was further adapted for the simultaneous measurement of emission and transmission by gating the acquisition process to synchronize with the scanning line position. The disadvantage of such a system is that it cannot readily be adapted for use with integrated, digital, camera computer acquisition systems due to the need to window the acquisition of emission data as the transmission source is scanned across the image. This requires access to either the analog or digital position signal prior to image formation which is often not the case in such integrated systems.

Recent developments in multi-detector systems have led to designs for the simultaneous measurement of transmission/emission data in one head with the remaining detectors acquiring only emission data. For a triangular configuration, in conjunction with the use of fan beam collimators, a line source at the focus of the collimator can be used to provide a measurement of the combined emission and transmission from one detector, the emission-only distribution coming from the remaining two detectors. For systems using cone beam collimators a point source can be placed at the focus of one collimator to provide the same combination of data[13,14]. Simultaneous measurements of emission and transmission are to be preferred to sequential measurements due to problems of realignment and patient movement. Systems using ring geometries, square detector arrays or two opposed detectors cannot readily be adapted for such simultaneous measurements.

Two detectors at right angles do permit attenuation measurements using static point or line, plane or scanning line sources depending on the collimation used.

Systems based on this geometry are currently under development by a number of manufacturers. The concept of a variable geometry system to provide two opposed detectors or two detectors at right angles offers significant advantages for general purpose applications. Fan and cone beam collimation may be used to increase resolution and sensitivity for brain applications whilst parallel collimation may be used for body imaging.

The incorporation of attenuation data is usually achieved by the use of iterative reconstruction methods[8]. Such reconstruction methods allow for the correction of the non-stationary resolution of the detector as well as allowing for estimates of the scatter distribution. For these reasons, iterative reconstruction methods are receiving increased attention, particularly as computers continue to become faster and cheaper.

*Scatter correction*

Scatter correction in SPET is a more difficult problem than attenuation since it is dependent on the radioactive distribution itself as well as the distribution of attenuation coefficients. Its effect can only adequately be compensated by the use of full 3-D iterative reconstruction methods which take these two components into account.

The effect of scatter is the degradation of contrast in the image. Volumes of zero activity concentration have an apparent concentration due to the scattered photons attributed as originating from that volume in the imaging process. The scatter distribution is known to be highly correlated with the primary distribution. This has led to the use of a modified linear attenuation coefficient to compensate for both attenuation and scatter. The decrease in contrast associated with the scattering process will influence the accuracy of edge detection algorithms. The majority of the scattered photons originate from structures surrounding and containing the radio-tracer such as the patient couch and the gamma camera detection system. The limited energy resolution of the scintillation detectors used in SPET leads to a poor discrimination of scattered and unscattered photons.

Estimates of the scatter contribution have been made using a number of different techniques. Many have been based upon the use of multiple pulse height analyser windows. As well as the primary photopeak one or more additional windows may be used to estimate the amount of scatter in the photopeak window[20,35]. Estimates have also been made directly from the photopeak data itself by convolution with an appropriate filter which is usually derived empirically[1,29].

All these techniques remain estimates and without a full iterative simulation of the imaging process utilizing the attenuation and emission data all scatter correction techniques are approximations.

The problems of the non-stationary finite detector response will also need to be addressed. Iterative techniques which model the system point spread function have been developed. Another area of development has been to use a high resolution anatomical image from either CT or MRI for the brain[22]. Following reconstruction the MRI or CT data is used to correct the SPET data for the partial volume effect. This may be an appropriate mechanism for use in the brain.

It is clear that the problems of attenuation and scatter are not solved at present for routine clinical application. It is essential that SPET techniques are developed to provide absolute activity quantification. Without this ability direct comparisons between centres and different instrumentation cannot readily be made. Systems manufacturers will develop transmission scanning capabilities which will be coupled to the development of statistically based iterative reconstruction methods. Methods for speeding these reconstruction methods are already in development and the continued development of computer processing power will make their application in clinical routine feasible.


## Discussion

Whilst there is a clear relationship between radiopharmaceutical and instrumentation development these must be viewed critically in relation to the clinical application. Two recent review articles have sought to put these developments into a clinical context both in the area of cerebral blood flow measurement[5] and neuroreceptor studies[4]. Both articles seek to address the need for stable and reproducible techniques if significant impact is to be made into clinical practice. The generation of control databases will require co-operation between many centres requiring a consensus on the methods of data acquisition and reconstruction.

The recent development of radiotracers has been concentrated upon ligands retained by the brain to produce an essentially static distribution and capable of being labelled with $^{99m}$Tc. This trend has led to systems often optimized for photon energies below 200 keV. There is thus now a feedback loop which concentrates further radiotracer development to this energy range in order to utilize the current range of detectors. Thallium in the form of $^{201}$Tl-chloride has become the focus for studies in oncology and in particular for the study of tumour recurrence and tumour staging. The low energy emissions from $^{201}$Tl are suitable for imaging with the current generation of brain SPET optimized systems. However, tracers labelled with $^{111}$In, $^{67}$Ga and $^{131}$I will not easily be imaged with systems optimized below 200 keV. $^{123}$I provides the only other tracer regularly used as a radiolabel for brain studies. $^{123}$I is currently the label of choice for the development of tracers for the study of neuroreceptors. Here the limited statistical accuracy obtained at permitted radiation doses is a major constraint to the quantification of these distributions especially where these studies present tracer distributions varying with time. $^{123}$I is a radionuclide which can readily be incorporated into these biological molecules, however, its dosimetry is poor and thus significant effort is being placed upon the replacement of $^{123}$I with $^{99m}$Tc.

Multi-headed SPET systems offer a substantial increase in tomographic volume sensitivity compared to a single rotating gamma camera. Depending on collimator type and collimator design parameters, better tomographic spatial resolution is achievable. For brain applications this gain in resolution is essential to improve quantification and delineation of important brain structures. For the multi-detector systems such as the SME-810 considerable further gains in tomographic volume sensitivity when expressed in terms of a single slice or centimetre of axial scan length are achieved, however, when considering the total volume of the brain these devices offer no significant gains over the multiple Anger gamma camera systems with fan or cone beam collimators.

Collimator choice is one of the most important factors that determine image quality in nuclear medicine. In agreement with others[8,33,34], we recommend the use of high resolution collimators for brain SPET. Fan beam collimators can further improve resolution and sensitivity[19,32]. The apparent system planar resolution improves by the magnification effect. Cone beam collimation will yield a higher sensitivity but requires a scanning trajectory that will yield sufficient sampling of the 3-D volume[13].

System stability is an essential pre-requisite for the multi-headed systems and considerable advances have been made to ensure accurate rotation of the device. Systems such as the CER-ESPECT system have the advantage of not moving the detector, only the collimator, thus leading to improved stability. Electrical stability is still a factor which can only be ascertained from extended observation of individual systems. Where multiple detectors have to remain stable with respect to each other the need for rapid and sensitive quality assurances measures is a paramount consideration in the choice of device. For some systems, stability may be obtained at the expense of scanning speed. Here, figures quoted for tomographic volume sensitivity must be interpreted with care since significant losses may result in clinical applications. The availability and use of continuous rotation modes provides optimization of tomographic volume sensitivity.

Improvements in detector technology have led to an increase in the energy resolution of all gamma camera systems. There still remains a significant difference in the energy resolution of systems. It is essential that the energy or pulse height window used for tomographic imaging is matched to the energy resolution of the system. Considerable improvements in contrast resolution in reconstructed data has been demonstrated by using either offset (20 per cent offset 3 per cent) or narrow (15 per cent) energy windows. These measures can produce improvements of between 5 and 10 per cent in grey to white matter ratios through the rejection of scatter. The use of a narrow window for systems with improved energy resolution does not significantly reduce the tomographic volume sensitivity. These improvements, coupled with optimized used of pulse height analyser window setting, have enabled dual isotope studies to be performed with $^{99m}$Tc and $^{123}$I.

For variable geometry systems, the user has to configure the detector during patient positioning to minimize the radius of rotation. This latter point raises the issue of reproducibility and measurement errors in patient populations. It is clear that changes in this parameter will impinge on the reconstructed image. Variable radii of rotation will change the effective resolution within an individual patient study and through the partial volume effect can considerably distort the radiotracer distribution from one study to the next. For repeat studies on different occasions it is essential that equivalent scanning conditions are used. From an analysis of the measurement of relative Ceretec uptake in different areas of the brain using both a single head detector and a fixed-geometry multi-detector system and the same reconstruction parameters, it has been shown that the range of values obtained in a control populations are significantly reduced when a fixed geometry system is used. These reduced value ranges will ultimately lead to better population discrimination and for this reason the use of fixed geometry systems is to be recommended, rather than variable geometry systems which rely on operator skills for optimal use. The need for a systematic approach cannot be overemphasized.

Improvements in resolution in space and energy need to be matched by improvements in acquisition parameters. The pixel size and the number of projections define the angular and spatial sampling, respectively. It is suggested that the finest acquisition matrix that could be practically employed should be used. The acquisition matrix need not be the same size as the reconstruction matrix, indeed it should be finer. In terms of pixel size, this depends on the camera field of view and the matrix size and should optimally be < FWHM (mm)/3. Thus this parameter can be matched to collimator choice and the clinical problem under investigation.

The tomographic process is not very sensitive to the number of angles employed, nor to whether 'step and shoot' or continuous rotation is employed, provided that the binning for continuous rotation is sufficiently fine. The angular sampling required is such that the circumferential arc traversed between projections, at the surface of the organ of interest, should be equal to the pixel size. For the brain this would indicate that for a 3 mm pixel size and a nominal brain diameter of 20 cm, there should be approximately 200 projections. Typically numbers of projections range from 64 to 128. In practice this represents a significant undersampling of the data. For the brain, improvements continue to be seen where angular sampling is decreased to 3° or less and these changes become more significant as spatial resolution increases. This is because the major improvements are seen at the periphery of the organ which is where the majority of the detailed structures reside in the brain.

Once the data has been acquired, a systematic analysis protocol must be adopted. It is necessary to decide on the appropriate reconstruction method. What reconstruction filter should be applied to improve resolution and or improve noise? Should scatter correction be applied? Should attenuation correction be applied?

Sampling theory states that the resolution and hence pixel size of the final reconstruction must be less than one-half of the size of the object to be detected. This implies that an appropriate window function must be used, that is the shape of the smoothing filter must be correctly chosen. This means primarily choosing the cut-off frequency of the window function, which for small objects should not be less than 0.5 of the Nyquist frequency. For larger objects, this could be reduced. These sampling recommendations apply also to the choice of slice thickness. Note that the filtering across slices changes the effective slice thickness, and also effective sensitivity and resolution. Since SPET is intrinsically 3-D, the filters used across slices should be similar to those used within slices, that is the shape of the filter should be isotropic in 3-D.

# References

1.      Axelsson, B., Msaki, P. & Israelsson, A. (1984): Subtraction of Compton scattered photons in single-photon emission computerized tomography. *J. Nucl. Med.* **25**, 490–494.

2.      Bailey, D.L., Hutton, B.F. & Walker, P.J. (1987): Improved SPECT using simultaneous emission transmission tomography. *J. Nucl. Med.* **28**, 844–851.

3.      Blokland, J.A.K., Reiber, J.H.C. & Pauwels, E.K.J. (1992): Quantitative analysis in single photon emission tomography. *Eur. J. Nucl. Med.* **19**, 47–61.

4.      Budinger, T.F. (1992): Critical review of PET, SPECT and neuroreceptor studies in schizophrenia. *J. Neural Transm. [Suppl]* **36**, 3–12.

5.      Ell, P.J. (1992): Mapping cerebral blood flow. *J. Nucl. Med.* **33**, 1843–1845.

6.      Evans, A.C., Beil, C., Marrett, S., Thompson, C.J. & Hakim, A. (1988): Anatomical-functional correlation using an adjustable MRI-based region of interest atlas with positron emission tomography. *J. Cereb. Blood Flow Metab.* **8**, 513–529.

7.      Evans, A.C., Marrett, S., Torrescorzo, J., Ku, S. & Collins, L. (1991): MRI–PET correlation in three dimensions using a volume-of-interest (VOI) atlas. *J. Cereb. Blood Flow Metab.* **11**, A69–A78.

8.      Fahey, F.H., Harkness, B.A., Keyes, J.W., Madsen, M.T., Battisti, C. & Zito, V. (1992): Sensitivity, resolution and image quality with a multi-head SPECT camera. *J. Nucl. Med.* **33**, 1859–1863.

9.      Fleming, J.S. (1989): A technique for using CT images in attenuation correction and quantification in SPECT. *Nucl. Med. Commun.* **10**, 83–97.

10.     Frey, E.C., Tsui, B.M.W. & Perry, R. (1992): Simultaneous acquisition of emission and transmission data for improved Thallium-201 cardiac SPECT imaging using a Technetium-99m transmission source. *J. Nucl. Med.* **33**, 2238–2245.

11.     Genna, S. & Smith, A.P. (1988): The development of ASPECT, an annular single crystal brain camera for high efficiency SPECT. *IEEE Trans. Nucl. Sci* **NS-35**, 654–658.

12.     George, M., Ring, H., Costa, D.C., Kouris, K., Jarritt, P.H. & Ell, P.J. (1991): *Neuroactivation and neuroimaging with SPET*. Heidelberg: Springer.

13.     Gullberg, G.T., Zeng, G.L., Christian, P.E., Datz, F.L. & Morgan, H.T. (1991): Cone beam tomography of the heart using SPECT. *Invest. Radiol.* **26**, 681–688.

14.     Gullberg, G.T., Zeng, G.L., Datz, F.L., Christian, P.E., Tung, C.-H., & Morgan, H.T. (1992): Review of convergent beam tomography in single photon emission tomography. *Phys. Med. Biol.* **37**, 507–534.

15.     Hawkes, D.J., Hill, D.L.G., Lehmann, E.D., Robinson, G.P. Maisey, M.N. & Colchester, A.C.F. (1990): Preliminary work on the interpretation of SPECT images with the aid of registered MR images and MR derived 3D neuro-anatomical atlas. In: *3D imaging in medicine*, eds K.H. Hoehne, S.M. Pizer & H. Fuchs, pp. 241–252. Berlin, Heidelberg, New York: Springer.

16. Hawkes, D.J., Robinson, L., Crossman, J.E., Sayman, H.B., Mistry, R., Maisey, M.N. & Spencer, J.D. (1991): Registration and display of the combined bone scan and radiograph in the diagnosis and management of wrist injuries. *Eur. J. Nucl. Med.* **18**, 752–756.

17. Hisada, K. (ed) (1991): *An atlas of second generation SPECT*. Maruzen Planning Network, Japan

18. Hoffman, E.J., Cutler, P.D., Digby, W.M. & Mazziotta, J.C. (1990): 3-D phantom to simulate cerebral blood flow and metabolic images for PET. *IEEE Trans, Nucl. Sci.* **37**, 616–620.

19. Jaszczak, R.J., Chang, L.T. & Murphy, P.H. (1979): Single photon emission computed tomography using multi-slice fan beam collimators. *IEEE Trans Nucl. Sci.* **26**, 610–618.

20. Jaszczak, R.J., Floyd, C.E. & Coleman, R.E. (1985): Scatter compensation techniques for SPECT. *IEEE Trans. Nucl. Sci.* **NS-32**, 786–793.

21. Kim, H.-J., Zeeberg, B.R., Fahey, F.H., Bice, A.N., Hoffman, E.J. & Reba, R.C. (1991): Three-dimensional SPECT simulations of a complex three-dimensional mathematical brain model and measurements of the three-dimensional brain phantom. *J. Nucl. Med.* **32**, 1923–1930.

22. Kim, H.-J., Zeeberg, B.R. & Reba, R.C. (1992): Compensation for three-dimensional detector response, attenuation and scatter in SPECT grey matter imaging using an iterative reconstruction algorithm which incorporates a high resolution anatomical image. *J. Nucl. Med.* **33**, 1225–1234.

23. Kimura, K., Hashikawa, K., Etani, H. *et al.* (1990): A new apparatus for brain imaging: a four-head rotating gamma camera single-photon emission computed tomograph. *J. Nucl. Med.* **31**, 603–609.

24. King, M.A., Long, D.T. & Brill, B.A. (1991): SPECT volume quantitation: influence of spatial resolution, source size and shape, and voxel size. *Med. Phys.* **18**, 1016–1024.

25. Kouris, K., Jarritt, P.H., Costa, D.C. & Ell, P.J. (1992): Physical assessment of the GE/CGR Neurocam and comparison to a single rotating gamma camera. *Eur. J. Nucl. Med.* **19**, 236–242.

26. Kuhl, D.E. & Edwards, R.Q. (1963): Image separation radioisotope scanning. *Radiology* **80**, 653.

27. Lee, K.H., Liu, H.T.H., Chen, D.C., Seigal, M.E. & Ballard, S. (1988): Volume calculation by means of SPECT: analysis of imaging acquisition and processing factors. *Radiology* **167**, 259–262.

28. Lim, C.B., Walker, R., Pinkstaff, C., *et al.* (1986): Triangular SPECT system for 3-D total organ volume imaging: performance results and dynamic imaging capability. *IEEE Trans. Nucl. Sci.* **33**, 501–504.

29. Ljunberg, M. & Strand, S.-E. (1990): Scatter and attenuation correction in SPECT using density maps and Monte Carlo simulated scatter functions. *J. Nucl. Med.* **31**, 1560–1567.

30. Madsen, M.T., Chang, W. & Hichwa, R.D. (1992): Spatial resolution and count density requirements in brain SPECT imaging. *Phys. Med. Biol.* **37**, 1625–1636.

31. Maisey, M.N., Hawkes, D.J. & Lukawiecke-Vydelingum, A.M. (1992): Synergistic imaging. *Eur. J. Nucl. Med.* **19**, 1002–1005.

32. Moore, S.C., Kouris, K. & Cullum, I. (1992): Collimator design for single photon emission tomography. *Eur. J. Nucl. Med.* **19**, 138–150.

33. Muehllehner, G. (1985): Effect of resolution improvement on required count density in ECT imaging: a computer simulation. *Phys. Med. Biol.* **30**, 163–173.

34. Mueller, S.P., Pollak, J.F., Kijewski, M.F. & Holman, B.L. (1986): Collimator selection for SPECT brain imaging: the advantage of high resolution. *J. Nucl. Med.* **27**, 1729–1738.

35. Ogawa, K., Harata, Y., Ichihara, T., Kubo, A. & Hashimoto, S. (1990): A new method for scatter correction in SPECT. *Med. Phys.* **17**, 518.

36. Smith, A.P. & Genna, S. (1989): Imaging characteristics of ASPECT. A single-crystal ring camera for dedicated brain SPECT. *J. Nucl. Med.* **30**, 796.

37. Stoddart H.F. & Stoddart, H.A. (1979): A new development in single gamma transaxial tomography – Union Carbide focused collimator scanner. *IEEE Trans. Nucl. Sci.* **26**, 2710–2712.

38. Stokely, E.M., Sveinsdottir, E., Lassen, N.A. & Rommer, P. (1980): A single photon dynamic computer assisted tomograph (DCAT) for imaging brain function in multiple cross sections. *J. Comput. Assist. Tomog.* **4**, 230–240.

39. Tan, P., Bailey, D.L., Hutton, B.F. *et al.* (1989): A moving line source for simultaneous transmission/emission SPECT. *J. Nucl. Med.* **30**, 964.

# Section IV
# RADIOPHARMACEUTICALS FOR BRAIN IMAGING

The selective characteristics of the blood–brain barrier (BBB) impose tight rules on the passage of molecules and solutes from the blood to the brain. Highly lipophilic and neutral substances diffuse freely into the brain cells, whilst other polar chemicals and ions do not cross the endothelial barrier. Ions and water are secreted into the cerebro-spinal fluid (CSF) via the choroid plexus in the lateral ventricles. Other chemicals may reach the astroglia and neurons after being carried through the brain endothelium with significant energy expenditure (active transport or facilitated transport).

Radiopharmaceuticals for brain imaging are not exempt from these rules. As has been mentioned in Chapter 2, some radiotracers ($^{99m}$Tc-pertechnetate, $^{99m}$Tc-DTPA, $^{99m}$Tc-glucoheptonate, $^{201}$Tl-thallous chloride, $^{67}$Ga-citrate) do not cross the intact BBB and are called conventional BBB tracers. They will all pass through a disrupted BBB with increased permeability, as happens in cases of infarct (stroke) and tumours (primary and/or secondary). On the contrary, other lipophilic and neutral radiopharmaceuticals (discussed later in this book) have been recently developed with the aim of obtaining images and measurements of brain functions. These include: the brain perfusion tracers ($^{99m}$Tc-HMPAO, $^{99m}$Tc-ECD, $^{99m}$Tc-MRP20) also known as regional cerebral blood flow (rCBF) agents, after $^{133}$Xe and others labelled with positron emitters, e.g. $^{15}$O-water, $^{15}$O-C dioxide, $^{11}$C-C dioxide etc.; the $^{18}$F-deoxyglucose to measure glucose metabolism; the tumour markers ($^{123}$I-iodomethyltyrosine, a single photon emitter; $^{11}$C-methionine and $^{18}$F-fluorodeoxyuridine, positron emitters); the neuroreceptor imaging tracers ($^{123}$I-iodobenzamide, $^{123}$I-QNB, $^{123}$I-dexetimide, $^{123}$I-iomazenil, single photon emitters and $^{11}$C- raclopride, $^{11}$C-N-methylspiperone, $^{11}$C-flumazenil, $^{11}$C-carfentanyl, positron emitters) and the precursors of neurotransmitters ($^{18}$F- dopa).

*New Trends in Nuclear Neurology and Psychiatry*, edited by D.C. Costa, G.F. Morgan and N. A. Lassen
© 1993 John Libbey & Company Ltd., pp. 65–84

# Chapter 5

# Radiopharmaceuticals for conventional blood–brain barrier and brain perfusion studies

G.F. Morgan[1] and D.C. Costa[2]

[1]*Amersham International plc, Amersham Place, Little Chalfont, Buckinghamshire, UK, and* [2]*Institute of Nuclear Medicine, University College of London, London, UK*

## I. Radiopharmaceuticals for conventional blood-brain barrier studies

### Introduction

With the advent of X-ray computerized tomography (CT scan) and more recently magnetic resonance imaging (MRI) the initial euphoria for conventional BBB tracers quickly disappeared. The decision to include them in this book is not only an historical one. In addition to this we believe that they still may play a role in the peripheral primary referral health centres, where CT scan and MRI are not easily available. This is emphasized by the long waiting lists and particularly the need for a quick diagnosis of brain metastases with a relatively high patient sensitivity. Even in a tertiary referral centre (University affiliated hospital), the occasional conventional BBB study is requested by oncologists/radiotherapists to confirm or otherwise the presence of brain metastases, particularly in elderly patients. Although comparison with MRI has never been established and will probably never be made, when compared to CT scans, conventional BBB radionuclide imaging with single photon emission tomography (SPET) showed concordant results in 81 per cent of 209 patients studied[17]. Furthermore the false positive rates for SPET and CT scan were respectively 0 per cent and 0.5 per cent, whilst the false negative rates were calculated respectively at 2.4 per cent and 6 per cent. To date, this similar sensitivity for the detection of metastatic brain disease between SPET and CT scan has never been challenged.

This technique may still be of great value in studying patients with claustrophobia and others reluctant to enter in a MRI tunnel.

In the late 1970s and early 1980s several reports demonstrated the superiority of SPET over planar imaging of the brain using conventional BBB tracers. The improvement in sensitivity of detection of lesions varied from 7 per cent to 20 per cent over that of planar scintigraphy (Table 1).

Another area where these conventional BBB tracers appear to play a singularly effective role is in the differentiation between post-irradiation necrosis and tumour recurrence. Both CT scan and MRI show little efficacy whilst the use of $^{201}$Tl has been reported as useful for the preoperative evaluation of patients with primary brain tumours[32] and highly sensitive in the detection of tumour recurrence and grading of intracranial tumours[3,30]. No $^{201}$Tl uptake is demonstrated in necrosis post- irradiation, oedematous tissue or normal cells[25].

Table 1. Reported improvement on sensitivity of detection of brain lesions with SPET over planar scintigraphy

| Author | Year | n (subjects) | Sensitivity gain (per cent) | Comments |
|---|---|---|---|---|
| Dendy et al.[10] | 1977 | 57 | 7 | Greater reporting confidence with SPET |
| Carrill et al.[7] | 1979 | 512 | 14 | Marked increase in true positive results with no change in the false positive rate |
| Ell et al.[17] | 1980 | 209 | 20 | Added sensitivity, improved lesion localization and reporting performance |
| Hill et al.[27] | 1980 | 200 | 10 | Improved sensitivity and specificity |
| Watson et al.[71] | 1980 | 238 | 0 | No significant and measurable benefit of SPET over plain scintigraphy |

## $^{99m}$Tc-pertechnetate

$^{99m}$Tc was discovered in 1938 by Seabourg & Segre[20]. However, its clinical utility was delayed until the development of the generator concept by the independent efforts of Richards & Harper in the early 1960s[44] made this radioisotope more accessible. Technetium is a second-row transition metal belonging to group VIIB, whose congeners are manganese (Mn) and rhenium (Re). It has an atomic number of 43 and although many radioisotopic forms have been isolated and identified there is no stable isotope of technetium known to occur naturally. Technetium, in common with many of the transition metals, will form stable complexes where the metal is present in a number of different oxidation states. Technetium complexes have been characterized where the oxidation state of the metal has varied from $-1$ to $+7$. The most stable oxidation states are $+7$ and $+4$. The pertechnetate ion ($TcO_4{}^-$) has the oxidation state of $+7$ for $^{99m}$Tc and is a very stable complex in solution. Pertechnetate is structurally similar to permanganate ($MnO_4{}^-$) and perrhenate ($ReO_4{}^-$). However, whilst the chemistry of pertechnetate and perrhenate shows strong similarities, permanganate differs markedly from the other two.

Although the chemistry of $^{99m}$Tc is complex and not fully understood, its almost ideal physical characteristics for gamma camera imaging (monoenergetic 140 keV gamma photons and 6 h physical half-life), in addition to its favourable radiation dosimetry, made it the radionuclide of choice for labelling newly developed molecules. It is readily available in a sterile and pyrogen-free solution of sodium pertechnetate, following elution from a $^{99}$Mo/$^{99m}$Tc generator. Once administered intravenously, the pertechnetate ion is taken up by secretory glands (thyroid, salivary, stomach, etc.) and is secreted into the CSF by the choroid plexus. This has been its major drawback for brain imaging. The administration of potassium perchlorate some 20 min before the injection is used to abolish the choroid plexus secretion and visualization, as well as uptake by the other glands[26].

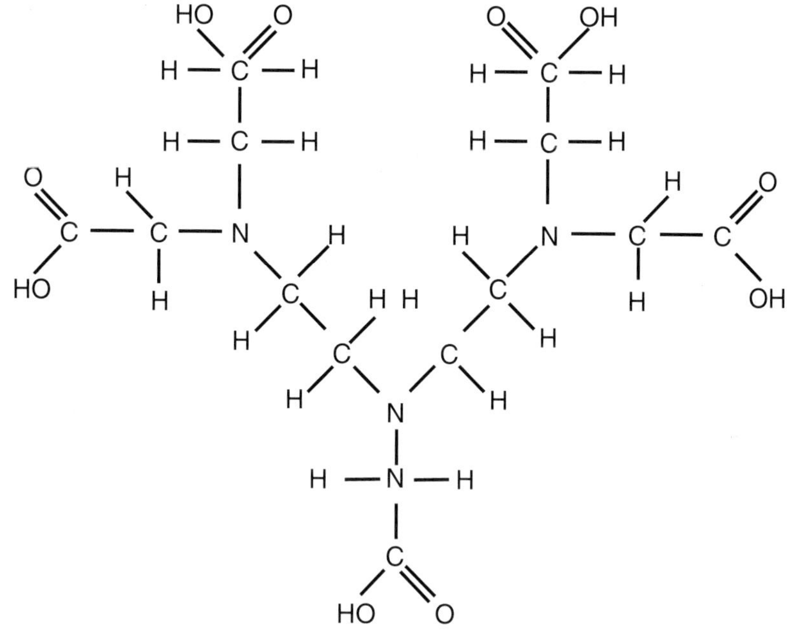

*Fig. 1. Chemical structure of diethylenetriamine pentaacetic acid (DTPA).*

Because the complex possesses an overall electrical charge, it will not cross the intact BBB. Its excretion is mainly through the kidneys and by passive diffusion into the bowel lumen.

With the increased availability of $^{99m}$Tc-DTPA and of $^{99m}$Tc-glucoheptonate, the pertechnetate ion, as sodium pertechnetate, fell into disuse.

## $^{99m}$Tc-diethylenetriamine pentaacetic acid($^{99m}$Tc- DTPA)

DTPA is an organic molecule (Fig. 1) which will chelate with technetium to form a stable, water soluble complex at physiological pH. $^{99m}$Tc-DTPA is prepared by reducing pertechnetate (TcO$_4$$^-$) with a suitable reducing agent in the presence of CaNa$_3$DTPA. Stannous (Sn$^{2+}$), in the chemical form SnCl$_2$2H$_2$O, is the most commonly used reductant in radiopharmaceutical preparations. The radiopharmaceutical is provided as a lyophilized kit containing the stannous reductant and upon reconstitution with pertechnetate in saline gives the desired $^{99m}$Tc-DTPA product with a more than 95 per cent yield. The complex remains stable and suitable for use for up to 6 h post-preparation.

After intravenous administration, it is distributed to the kidneys where it is mainly excreted by glomerular filtration. Otherwise it remains partially intravascular (free and bound to plasma proteins) and labels mainly the extravascular and extracellular water space. The renal excretion is significantly faster than $^{99m}$Tc (pertechnetate). This offers an advantage for brain imaging. Studies of breakdown of the BBB can be carried out earlier than with pertechnetate and the target-to-background ratio improves due to the quicker washout from the blood stream. In addition, another advantage over $^{99m}$TcO$_4$$^-$ is the non-visualization of the choroid plexus. The administration of potassium perchlorate in advance of the injection becomes unnecessary.

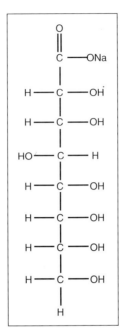

*Fig. 2. Chemical structure of sodium glucoheptonate.*

### 99mTc-glucoheptonate

Sodium glucoheptonate (GH) is a complex based on the configuration of sugars (Fig. 2). The radiopharmaceutical, similar to [99m]Tc-DTPA, is supplied as a freeze-dried preparation for reconstitution with pertechnetate. [99m]Tc-GH is not metabolized and is excreted in the urine without any modification of its chemical structure. The renal excretion is by a combination of glomerular filtration and tubular secretion, which gives rise to a more rapid fall of blood levels when compared to pertechnetate and [99m]Tc-DTPA. In addition, after intravenous administration, it rapidly equilibrates in the extracellular space with little binding to plasma proteins. Consequently, imaging with glucoheptonate may be performed earlier after injection than with [99m]Tc-DTPA and pertechnetate. Furthermore the contrast between lesion (glioblastomas, meningiomas, abscesses and metastases) uptake and background radiation is higher allowing for better lesion definition[58], particularly when SPET is used.

Whilst the first studies indicated that early plain images with glucoheptonate offered little advantage over pertechnetate[72,57], there is no doubt that using SPET there are advantages on scanning earlier (60 min post-injection) than later (90–120 min post-injection), particularly due to higher photon yields. This is highly beneficial for the reconstruction algorithm. It has already been shown (Table 1) that sensitivity of lesion detection is significantly improved by the use of SPET.

The initial studies have interestingly shown glucoheptonate to be better than pertechnetate in cases of intracranial tumours (primary or secondary), whilst secondaries in the skull and scalp could not be well visualized. This may indicate that different mechanisms[72] preside over the uptake of glucoheptonate and pertechnetate. Others[74,56] have reported on the uptake of glucoheptonate in acute myocardial infarction, an additional feature in favour of different uptake mechanisms.

[99m]Tc-glucoheptonate, due to its faster excretion, higher lesion-to-background radioactivity ratio

(obtained earlier) and similar costs in comparison to pertechnetate and DTPA, appears at present to be, ideally, the conventional BBB radiotracer of choice. As with $^{99m}$Tc-DTPA there is no need for the administration of potassium perchlorate in advance of the injection. Choroid plexuses are not visualized.

### $^{201}$Tl-thallous chloride

The main clinical application of $^{201}$Tl has been in the study of myocardial perfusion under stress and at rest. Discovered as early as 1861, thallium was introduced into the nuclear medicine clinical armamentarium as late as 1975[39].

It is produced by bombarding the isotope $^{203}$Tl in an accelerator (cyclotron) according to the reaction – $^{203}$Tl(p,3n) $^{201}$Pb. Subsequently, $^{201}$Pb decays to $^{201}$Tl with a half-life of 9.4 h. The final product is defined according to the trace amounts of $^{200}$Tl, $^{202}$Tl and $^{201}$Pb present in the final material. After irradiation with protons (35–45 MeV), the natural thallium target is dissolved in a mineral acid, and $^{201}$Pb is isolated by ion-exchange. The radionuclides of lead are absorbed into another ion-exchange column and enough time is allowed for $^{201}$Pb to decay (by electron capture) to $^{201}$Tl which is eluted as $^{201}$Tl-thallous chloride. Other options for thallium separation are available and may be used instead of the one above described.

$^{201}$Tl decays to $^{201}$Hg by electron capture with a half-life of 73.1 h. Two gamma photons are emitted with energies of 135 keV and 167 keV. Their abundance is however poor, reported as 3 per cent and 10 per cent respectively. Nevertheless, $^{201}$Hg produces X-rays of 68 to 80 keV with a reported frequency of 94.5 photons per 100 $^{201}$Tl atom disintegrations. These are the photons used for imaging with $^{201}$Tl.

After intravenous administration as thallous chloride $^{201}$Tl is distributed to the myocardium, skeletal muscle, liver, spleen, kidneys and gut according to the distribution of blood flow. In the past the uptake mechanism has been related to the sodium–potassium pump. However, there is now sufficient knowledge to make us believe that the cellular uptake of $^{201}$Tl is still more complicated and may depend on several factors rather than the ionic pump to be taken up by cells. It is well accepted that two main factors preside over the $^{201}$Tl uptake: blood flow and metabolic rate.

Very recently it has been reported that $^{201}$Tl is able to demonstrate brain tumours[3,30,32] as well as other tracers, including positron emitters like $^{18}$F-FDG[23,28], and it seems to be particularly useful in the differential diagnosis between tumour recurrence and post-irradiation necrosis[8,59].

### $^{67}$Ga-gallium citrate

There are two radioisotopes of gallium available for medical use as radionuclide imaging agents. One, $^{68}$Ga, is a positron emitter with a half-life of just 68 min and available from a generator – germanium-68 – gallium-68. In this generator, $^{68}$Ge in concentrated HCl is neutralized in EDTA solution and absorbed on the plastic or glass column of the generator. $^{68}$Ga may be eluted from this column with 0.005 M of EDTA solution. The resultant radiopharmaceutical may then be used for brain tumour imaging with PET. The other available radioisotope is $^{67}$Ga. It is an accelerator (cyclotron) produced radionuclide, obtained by the bombardment of a zinc target with protons, following the reaction –$^{67}$Zn(p,n)$^{67}$Ga-. The gallium is separated from the target and complexed with citrate to produce $^{67}$Ga-gallium citrate in sterile solution with a pH of 6–7. It decays by electron capture with a half-life of approximately 78 h, emitting three useful gamma photons. Their energies and abundance are as follows: 93 keV – 38 per cent, 185 keV – 24 per cent and 300 keV – 16 per cent. Another much less important gamma emission is the 394 keV with an abundance of only 4 per cent, and therefore of limited clinical value.

[67]Ga is commonly found in the +3 oxidation state only, and after intravenous injection quickly binds to iron-transporting proteins in the blood, particularly transferrin. Its circulating blood levels fall according to a multiple compartmental model. There are at least three well-defined rates of disappearance from the blood: (a) 50 per cent of the administered dose falls with a 9 min half-life, (b) a second rate of fall is observed immediately afterwards with a half-life of 2 h, and finally (c) the remaining activity (10 per cent of the injected dose) has a blood half-life of 48 h.

Renal cortex, liver, spleen, lachrymal and salivary glands, lactating breast, bone marrow, bowel and lymph nodes are amongst the organs usually considered to show [67]Ga uptake in normals at different times post-injection. Its excretion is via renal (10 per cent of the administered activity in 24 h ) and bowel routes (10 per cent over the first week).

Abnormal uptake is seen in inflammatory/infectious processes and tumours without any significant specificity. However, it has been considered as a good marker of lymph node involvement in patients with lymphoma and particularly the Hodgkin type. In addition, it has regained an important role in clinical nuclear medicine with the increasing frequency of acquired immunodeficiency syndrome (AIDS) and the need for localizing abdominal, thoracic and intracranial granulomas and tumours. Interestingly, it is not taken up by the granulomas of Kaposi's sarcoma.

**Tumour recurrence *vs* necrosis post-irradiation: radionuclides for tumour brain imaging**

There are three main therapeutic means to deal with brain tumours: surgery, radiotherapy and chemotherapy. Although these are reasonably effective, clinical deterioration due to either recurrence of the tumour or radiation necrosis in the radiotherapy field[43] is not rare. High-resolution structural imaging methodology available (CT scan, MRI and cerebral angiography) is unable to provide clear differentiation between these conditions. Either tumour recurrence or radiation necrosis may show enhancement when using contrast enhancing agents[5,18].

The most likely tool to assist in the distinction between metabolic active tumour (primary or recurrence) and post-irradiation necrotic tissue is the radioisotopic method due to its physiological behaviour. Radioactive diiodofluorescin[47] was the first radiotracer reported to differentiate normal from malignant tissues using the properties of the cold molecule fluorescin[46].

The introduction of [18]F-2-deoxyglucose (FDG)[55] to measure the degree of cerebral tissue glucose utilization originated a new path for the metabolic imaging of brain tumours. Based on Otto Warburg's[70] suggestion that tumours have higher rates of aerobic glycolysis (lactate production) with increasing degree of malignancy, several groups around the world have been using FDG and PET to grade primary tumours *in vivo*[13] and distinguish between tumour recurrence and post-irradiation necrosis[23,65].

Other tracers labelled with positron emitters (e.g. [18]F, [11]C or [13]N) have been suggested for the evaluation of brain tumours. They include sugar derivatives, amino acids, putrescine and receptor ligands. Amongst them the most promising appears to be the amino acid [11]C-methionine[51]. Thirty-six patients with cerebral tumours of different grades were studied demonstrating good correlation with histopathological grades obtained from multiple biopsies. In 23 cases delineation of the tumour was more accurate with PET and [11]C-methionine than with CT scan.

Unfortunately, the large experience of some PET users who carried out more than 1000 studies over the last decade cannot be extended to the majority of neurosurgical and oncological centres[14]. It is necessary to spread their ideas widely across the different levels of medical care in the community. This seems to be the major function of SPET. Indeed, the 'features of the "ideal" PET tracer for brain tumours' so carefully and elegantly described by Di Chiro[14] might be translated into 'features of the "ideal" SPET tracer for brain tumours', as follows:

(1) A clear rationale for the choice of a new tracer is desirable;

(2) Uptake in the tumour should be relatively independent of the status of the blood–brain barrier;

(3) Tracer retention in the tumour should be long enough to allow SPET studies to be carried out;

(4) The degree of tumour uptake should be correlated with the grade of the tumour, irrespective of the intimate uptake mechanism, and should permit the differentiation between tumour recurrence and radiation necrosis, post-operative sclerosis and non-viable components of the tumour (e.g. necrosis, cysts) distinctively from foci of aggressive tumour;

(5) There should be a good correlation between the tumour uptake of the tracer and the clinical outcome, in addition to the histopathological findings;

(6) The purity of the radiopharmaceutical and the resolution of the scanner should be adequate, giving enough contrast between grey and white matter, as well as between cortical and subcortical structures;

(7) Tested quantitative reliability should be available to support individual cases and to permit analysis of groups;

(8) Adequate reference areas should be chosen, taking into account the distribution of the tracer used;

(9) The reader should be experienced and skilled;

(10) Assessment of radiotracer capabilities should be based on a reasonable number of cases, certainly more than 20.

With these in mind, a review of the recent literature demonstrates that one tracer has been already showing a well-defined potential for the differential diagnosis of tumour recurrence and post-irradiation necrosis, [201]Tl as thallous chloride[59], whilst another, [123]I-L-AMT(3-iodo-alpha-methyl-L-tyrosine) is under research as an amino acid labelled with a single photon emitter. The former, [201]Tl, is a useful SPET radiotracer to assess brain tumours, either preoperatively or postoperatively, searching for recurrence or neoplastic residua. It differentiates between low and high grade tumours[32,45]. Low grade gliomas show low or no uptake of [201]Tl, in contrast to high grade gliomas which always demonstrate marked increase of the tracer concentration in the tumour compared to normal brain tisssue[45]. However, care should be taken due to the possible uptake of [201]Tl in brain abscesses[34]. In this single particular case, the [201]Tl uptake may have been due to the presence of intensive reactive gliosis and endothelial proliferation observed around the abscess. Brain perfusion studied with HMPAO and SPET depicted a large area of impaired (no HMPAO concentration) perfusion corresponding to the abscess and surrounding oedema. The combination of [201]Tl and brain perfusion SPET with HMPAO may prove to be the step forward in the evaluation of brain tumours pre- and postsurgery, as well as in the distinction between tumour recurrence and post-irradiation necrosis. In fact, this approach was used in a group of 15 consecutive patients with suspected recurrence of high grade glioma post-irradiation, seven with solid tumour confirmed with biopsy and eight with simple reactive post-irradiation changes on biopsy. All the seven patients with confirmed foci of solid tumour had increased [201]Tl uptake, classified as moderate in three and high in four. Five of the eight patients with no tumour had moderate [201]Tl uptake. The most discriminative power was obtained by the combination of [201]Tl and HMPAO uptake patterns. All but one of the patients with no tumour showed significant decreases of the HMPAO concentration in the abnormal structure. All the seven patients with tumour recurrence had either similar or increased HMPAO uptake, compared to normal brain tissue[59]. This novel approach deserves further evaluation using a larger study sample.

**Cerebral blood volume and haematocrit**

The importance of studying regional cerebral blood volume was for the first time emphasized by Gibbs *et al.* in 1984[21] when evaluating with PET the cerebral perfusion reserve in patients with carotid artery occlusion. A small reduction in regional cerebral blood flow was seen in some patients who presented with marked increases of the regional cerebral blood volume. Applying this methodology to the study of patients before and after EC–IC (external carotid–internal carotid) bypass the same group[22] has demonstrated that the predominant effect of surgery was to decrease regional cerebral blood volume.

The investigation of regional cerebral blood and plasma volume with SPET may be carried out by means of respectively labelled red blood cells and human serum albumin, that remain mainly intravascular. Red blood cells may be labelled with $^{99m}$Tc-pertechnetate after treatment with stannous chloride either *in vivo* or *in vitro*. Human serum albumin is usually labelled with $^{99m}$Tc-pertechnetate and in cases of combined studies with red blood cells it may be labelled with $^{123}$I.

Knapp *et al.*[33] described a method for the assessment of cerebral perfusion reserve by combining SPET with a perfusion tracer ($^{99m}$Tc-HMPAO) with red blood cell imaging. If one combines labelled red blood cells with labelled human serum albumin within the same SPET study, it is possible to determine the regional cerebral haematocrit, which is important for the cerebral autoregulation of blood flow and oxygen metabolism. Nowadays, activation protocols, particularly using physiological and/or pharmacological interventions (vasodilators, e.g. acetazolamide or adenosine) are favoured, instead of measures of regional blood or plasma volume.

## II. Radiopharmaceuticals for brain perfusion studies

**Introduction**

Radiopharmaceuticals for brain perfusion studies give insight into the regional blood flow (perfusion) status and the underlying function of areas or structures within the brain, making this technique a complementary tool to structural or anatomical neuroimaging. Used in conjunction with single photon emission tomography (SPET) cameras, functional brain SPET is establishing a role in clinical patient management and promises to become an integral part of routine clinical work-up for patients suffering from neurological and psychiatric disorders.

Quantification of global cerebral blood flow was first reported in the literature by Kety & Schmidt[31] over 40 years ago. Using nitrous oxide, it was possible to calculate blood flow, oxygen and glucose consumption in the whole brain but it was impossible to determine the function in selected areas of the brain. This latter aim was achieved in 1961 by Ingvar & Lassen[29] using the radioisotope $^{85}$Kr, later to be replaced by $^{133}$Xe. Following intracarotid injection of a saline solution of the gas, they plotted the rate of disappearance of the tracer from specific regions of interest, by the use of multiple probes arranged around the head. Intracarotid injection (an invasive and potentially morbid technique) was superseded by inhalation or intravenous administration of $^{133}$Xe and the measurement of cerebral blood flow in selected regions of the brain was available in the routine practice of nuclear medicine. The use of $^{133}$Xe and head probes became a regular tool for assessment of cerebral cortex rCBF, particularly because of its suitability for bedside measurements. However, information on blood flow to deeper structures in the brain was (and still is) difficult to obtain accurately even when tomographic (SPET) devices were used. This is due to the radionuclidic and physical properties of $^{133}$Xe which are not ideal when used in conjunction with currently available SPET technology. $^{133}$Xe-SPET lacks the contrast and spatial resolution which can be achieved with $^{99m}$Tc and $^{123}$I-labelled tracers. Thus a xenon analogue was required with the same biological and/or pharmacological characteristics but better imaging properties.

The remainder of this chapter will consider the history of development of brain perfusion agents suitable for SPET imaging and will discuss three classes of tracer in some detail; neutral thallium complexes, iodinated amines and neutral technetium complexes. The development of radiopharmaceuticals for PET imaging are outside of the scope of this chapter.

**Characteristics of a radiopharmaceutical for studying brain perfusion**

The primary requirement of a brain perfusion tracer is that the molecule will freely pass the BBB and distribute in proportion to regional blood flow. This is often referred to as 'the chemical microsphere'. There are two general mechanisms for transport across the BBB (which is required by definition to act as a barrier for foreign substances passing from the bloodstream into the brain), these are active membrane transport and passive diffusion. The first mechanism is highly structure dependent, relying upon molecular recognition of binding sites on protein carrier molecules, the latter mechanism is the one most commonly encountered in radiopharmaceutical drug design and is governed by some simple physico-chemical rules related to molecular size, weight, charge and overall lipophilicity (lipid solubility). Delivery of the tracer to the brain can be affected by any of these parameters and several studies have been published showing the relationships that exist between brain extraction and lipophilicity[16,53], molecular weight[41] and protein binding[42].

A second requirement of the radiopharmaceutical is that it will be efficiently extracted from the blood into neuronal tissue and will remain trapped for a period of time suitable for good SPET acquisition (20–60 min). A substance that freely diffuses across the BBB in one direction will backwash unless there is a trapping mechanism of some chemical/biochemical nature that prevents the back-diffusion out of the brain. The scientific literature is scattered with examples of radiolabelled tracers that cross the BBB freely in both directions – these will not serve a useful purpose in neuroimaging until gamma camera technology can acquire high quality SPET images within timescales that equate to the wash-in/wash-out of these tracers.

Iodoantipyrine, an iodinated amine, was the first molecule reported in the literature as a brain perfusion tracer in humans. It had similar behaviour to $^{133}$Xe. After distribution according to the regional cerebral blood flow, $^{123}$I-iodoantipyrine back-diffused rapidly from the brain into the blood[64]. The absence of a trapping mechanism inside the brain continued to be a significant drawback as the residence time in the brain of these tracers ($^{133}$Xe and $^{123}$I-iodoantipyrine) was too short to allow SPET imaging with the existing SPET technology. The first published paper to describe a trapping mechanism in the brain came in 1980 from Kung & Blau[36]. They reported on two diamines, MOSE and PIPSE (Fig. 3) labelled with the radionuclide $^{75}$Se. This mechanism has become known as the pH shift phenomenon. The trapping mechanism was attributed to the $pK_a$ of basic amines by the lower pH in brain neuronal tissue (7.0) compared to the pH of blood (7.4). After crossing the BBB, the amino group on the ligands pick up a proton at the intracellular pH of 7.0–7.15 and acquire a formal positive charge. A charged molecule will not passively back-diffuse across the BBB and is therefore trapped. It is now accepted that this explanation of the trapping mechanism may be an oversimplification. These tracers have not been tested in humans and because of the poor dosimetry and radiation characteristics (decays by electron capture with a $t_{1/2}$ of 119.8 days) of $^{75}$Se, they were never developed. The emphasis then shifted to the design of a radiopharmaceutical containing a radionuclide with better imaging characteristics that would be retained in the brain. pH shift is only one of a number of possible mechanisms that can result in a tracer being trapped in the brain, examples of others being

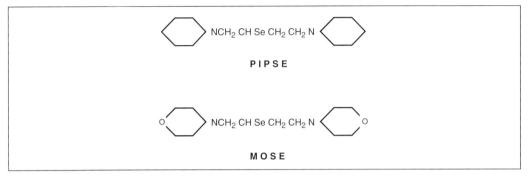

Fig. 3. Structure of PIPSE and MOSE.

specific binding to proteins or receptors, non-specific binding to proteins, intracellular interactions or hydrolysis.

## Neutral [201]Tl complexes

Diethyldithiocarbamate (DDC) (Fig. 4a) is a well-known chemical scavenger for heavy metal toxins in the body and has been used in detoxification from heavy metal (e.g. thallium) poisoning. However, clinical reports that this treatment occasionally lead to increased neurological symptoms suggested that the resulting Tl-DDC complex was crossing the BBB.

Biodistribution studies of [201]Tl-DDC were reported by de Bruine et al. [6] in rabbits and showed 1.46 per cent injected dose in the brain 25–45 min p.i., remaining stable for up to 1 h. Further animal work in rats and volunteer human studies established the high per cent injected dose in the whole brain (3.68 and 4.32 respectively) with slow wash-out of activity from the human brain (0.3 per cent loss of radioactivity/hour) compared to the faster wash-out observed with lesser primates.

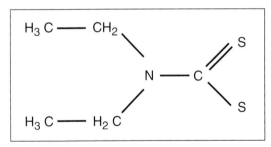

Fig. 4a. DDC (diethyldithiocarbamate).

In an autoradiographic comparison with [123]I-IMP and [14]C-iodoantipyrine, Lear et al. [38] showed that regional cerebral blood flow patterns of [201]Tl-DDC underestimated rCBF in low flow regions when compared with [14]C-IAP, taken as the gold standard of blood flow. A similar underestimation was found with [123]I-IMP and therefore [201]Tl-DDC was considered to distribute in the brain according to regional perfusion. Unlike [123]I-IMP, there was no asso-

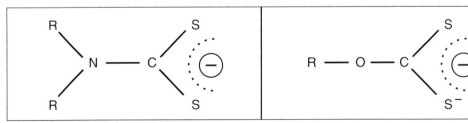

Fig. 4b. General formula of the dialkyldithio-carbamates, showing the coordinating group.

Fig. 4c. General formula of the xanthates.

ciated lung activity and peak brain uptake was reached in 90 s p.i. Image quality was compromised because of the 80 keV imaging photon and long half-life of $^{201}$Tl (73 h). A cross-over study with $^{99m}$Tc-HMPAO, involving 18 acute stroke patients, was reported by Van Royen[66] and image quality was recorded as being 'definitely better' for $^{99m}$Tc.

$^{201}$Tl-DDC is not commercially available and consequently must be prepared 'in house'. Its preparation however is simple, and forms a 1:1 complex which is stable at neutral and high pH and decomposes at low pH. Although the trapping mechanism within the brain is not elucidated, it may well reflect some acid-induced decomposition of the Tl-DDC complex. The disadvantage for $^{201}$Tl as a potential radioisotope in neuroimaging is its poor photon flux resulting in (relatively) poor image resolution and attenuation from the deeper lying structures compared to the more optimal imaging characteristics of $^{99m}$Tc or $^{123}$I. However the stability of $^{201}$Tl-DDC means that the radiopharmaceutical can be ready for injection 24 h a day.

Only DDC has been reported in the literature as a co-ordinating ligand although any dialkyldithiocarbamate (Fig. 4b) would complex in the same way (the co-ordinating group being the dithiodicarboxylate). An increase in alkyl chain length from two carbons to three or more would open up interesting structure distribution comparisons of brain uptake *vs* octanol:water partition coefficient (the indicator of lipophilicity). Neutral technetium complexes of DDC and aliphatic analogues have been reported in the literature by Ballinger *et al.*[2] The complexes are poorly characterized but appear to have some uptake and retention in the rabbit brain. There is no human data.

## $^{123}$I iodinated amines

There are several amines that play a central role in brain function. They are pharmacologically active, affecting the transport and uptake of brain metabolites and rates of synthesis and metabolism. It is likely that in neurological disorders amine kinetics and function are altered and therefore an indication of diseased state could be given by mapping amine function. The chemical structure of these naturally occurring amines is often suitable for iodination since they contain an aryl group, distal to the pharmacologically active site or recognition unit and therefore radioiodination with a radioisotope such as $^{123}$I could facilitate this mapping.

An iodinated diamine, developed by Kung *et al.*[37] theoretically took advantage of the pH difference between blood and brain – the 'pH shift phenomenon' previously described. However, a difference of 0.4 pH units between blood and intracellular brain space cannot account alone for the high first pass extraction efficiency and retention that was observed with HIPDM (and IMP described below). Brain uptake of HIPDM,[$^{123}$I]*N,N,N'*-trimethyl-*N'*-[2-hydroxy-3-methyl-5-iodobenzyl]-1,3-propanediamine, in humans was rapid and in the order of 4–5 per cent of the injected dose. Retention of the tracer was good, with steady state reported in the brain up to 4 h p.i. HIPDM is extracted by the lungs on first pass and slowly clears from there to the brain. Despite the positive features of HIPDM as a brain perfusion tracer, the rate of release from the lungs was considered too slow to warrant developing HIPDM as a commercial product.

In an attempt to mimic the biological activity of the amphetamines, a comprehensive study by Winchell *et al.* looked at 40 iodoarylalkylamines. This study made a valuable contribution to the early understanding of the influences of lipophilicity, stereochemistry and functional group placement on biological activity (distribution). The three classes of compounds studied were iodoanilines, iodobenzamines and iodophenethylamines, all structurally similar to amphetamine. In rats, 34 of the 40 iodinated ligands showed higher brain uptake and better brain-to-blood activity ratios than Winchell's gold standard, $^{123}$I-iodoantipyrine[73]. Differences in brain uptake and blood/brain ratios were observed within the same class by altering the placement of the

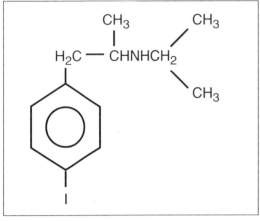

*Fig. 5. IMP.*

iodine from *ortho-* to *meta-* to *para-*positioning with respect to the amino functional group. Similarly, differences in biological activity were noticed between *R-* and *S-*isomers. Of the three separate ligand classes under study, the phenylalkylamines showed the most promising biological results and were developed further.

One derivative (Fig. 5) was selected for further study, because of its best biological characteristics in rats, *N*-$\alpha$-methylethyl-*p*-iodoamphetamine (IMP) now known commercially as Spectamine®. Following intravenous injection, IMP accumulates in the brain and distributes according to regional perfusion. Passage across the BBB was thought initially to be active transport through amine recognition, but it is now presumed to be passive diffusion, influenced by lipophilic partition coefficients and pH gradients. As with HIPDM, the tracer is initially sequestered in the lungs. IMP is released more rapidly from the lungs than HIPDM and the maximum activity that accumulates in the brain is higher for IMP (7 per cent of the injected dose) than for HIPDM (4 per cent i.d.). IMP was therefore a more suitable radiopharmaceutical to develop as a commercial product. The trapping mechanism in the brain is unknown. Several theories have been advanced, including the pH shift, amine metabolism and non-specific binding to amine-binding sites. Mori *et al.*[50] demonstrated saturable binding of [125]I-IMP in rat brains to high density non-specific binding sites where the affinity of IMP for these binding sites appeared to be enhanced with respect to the uniodinated ligand. It is however most likely that it is not one rate-limiting factor that determines the retention of these tracers in the brain but a number of contributing elements which include pH gradient, lipophilicity and non-specific binding sites.

The kinetics of uptake of IMP are considered near ideal. Quantification of brain uptake in the monkey showed a flow dependency. Kuhl[35] demonstrated that as blood flow increased from 33 ml/100 g/min to 66 ml/100 g/min, the extraction efficiency fell from 92 per cent to 74 per cent. It should be noted that there was an associated fall in arterial blood pH from 7.35 to 7.10 and this may therefore represent a diffusion limitation or pH effect or contribution of both factors. The same workers investigated kinetics in humans and showed that after i.v. injection, IMP is nearly completely removed on first pass through the brain. Steady state is reached after 5 min and the distribution, which is proportional to regional blood flow, remains almost constant for 1 h post-injection. Differential wash-out of the tracer from different regions of the brain means that delayed SPET acquisition may not produce the same distribution pattern as early SPET images and the recommended imaging time is 20 min to 1 h post-injection. Work by Greenberg and co-workers[24] confirmed the use of IMP as a CBF tracer by a validation study comparing [123]I-IMP and [15]O-H$_2$O. They concluded that under physiological conditions, IMP was a quantitative CBF tracer.

The quantification model for regional perfusion developed by Kuhl required sequential arterial blood sampling[35], an invasive technique which would preclude its regular use in the clinical setting. A quantification method has been recently published by Takeshita *et al.*[62] that requires arterial blood sampling at one time point and monitoring of the lung time-activity curve. rCBF values of 72 and 55 ml/100 mg/min were reported for the cortex and the brain hemisphere. These values were in good agreement with published data.

Initially, IMP was hindered as a radiopharmaceutical because of the availability and quality of the iodine. [123]I produced from a [124]Te target through the (p,2n) process contained significant amounts of [124]I which interfered with image quality and had implications for dosage regimens. With improved iodine production methods now in manufacturing practice or awaiting approval [[127]I (p,5n) and [124]Xe (p,2n)] radioisotopically purer iodine is achieved and the earlier objections are removed. Availability remains an inherent problem of [123]I-labelled radiopharmaceuticals but despite the logistical problems of patient scheduling with an [123]I radiopharmaceutical, IMP is widely used in certain regions of the world, notably Japan.

Recently, the use of a dual isotope protocol with [123]I-IMP has been validated by Devous and co-workers[11,12] which exploits the gamma photon energy differences between [123]I and [99m]Tc. [99m]Tc-HMPAO is injected under normal resting conditions – this is the baseline scan. An activation procedure or pharmacological stress agent (e.g. acetazolamide injection) is administered, followed by an injection of [123]I-IMP. Because of the *in vivo* stability (no redistribution, minimal wash-out) of [99m]Tc-HMPAO in the brain, simultaneous acquisition of [99m]Tc and [123]I gives an accurate map of the brain perfusion before and after the stress procedure. Furthermore, the two images are anatomically registered to one another. Because of the close proximity of the two gamma photon energies (140 and 159 keV), dual isotope imaging with [99m]Tc and [123]I is not possible with gamma cameras whose energy resolution is greater than 10 per cent FWHM.

## [99m]Tc brain perfusion tracers

The story of a brain perfusion tracer labelled with [99m]Tc is a celebration of the serendipitous method of drug development. Unlike iodinated molecules, where the iodine is assumed not to adversely affect the distribution of the parent ligand, most technetium radiopharmaceuticals exhibit biological behaviour that is totally different to the uncomplexed ligand. There are inevitably exceptions to both these rules but in general, biodistribution of a technetium radiopharmaceutical cannot be predetermined by knowledge of the biodistribution of the uncoordinated ligand. Thus the design of a brain perfusion tracer has to start with consideration of the basic rules in Table 2 and use knowledge of the inorganic chemistry of technetium to arrive at the desired biological end-point.

In the following paragraphs, aspects of overall complex charge, lipid solubility, molecular weight and stereochemistry will be discussed as they affect biological activity and examples will be drawn from the published literature of both commercially available preparations and those products still in development

The starting point of any technetium radiopharmaceutical is sodium pertechnetate. This is the chemical form of [99m]Tc as eluted from a commercial generator and is the chemical form that is added to any commercial 'cold kit'. As pertechnetate, technetium is present in its highest oxidation state (VII) and is thermodynamically stable. In order to promote complex formation with a ligand, a reducing agent is required which will reduce the oxidation state of the technetium from (VII) to a lower value which will stabilize in the presence of the ligand. As the

*Table 2. Physico-chemical rules governing passive diffusion across the blood-brain barrier*

| Feature | Range |
| --- | --- |
| Lipid soluble | Log P 0.9–2.5 |
| Moderate size | M.Wt < 400 Daltons |
| Overall charge | Neutral |
| Protein binding | Affected by lipophilicity/M.Wt |

oxidation state is altered, so is the formal charge on the metal ion. For example, as Tc(V), the metal ion bears a theoretical 5+ charge, as Tc(I), the metal ion bears a theoretical 1+ charge. The relevance of the charge on the metal ion becomes clear in drug design when attempting to synthesize a technetium complex having an overall neutral charge, i.e. the charge on the central metal core is cancelled out by the charge of the co-ordinating ligand. In practice, the reducing agent used commercially to produce technetium radiopharmaceuticals is stannous chloride (or fluoride) and the reduced technetium state that has been best characterized as Tc(V) with a mono-oxo or di-oxo core. This results in an overall charge on the technetium core of +3 and +1 respectively.

In the early 1980s two different ligand classes were being extensively investigated – the dioximes and the diaminodithiols. In 1984, Troutner *et al.*[63] published the *in vitro* radiopharmaceutical characteristics of 3,3′-(1,3-propanediyldiimino)bis-(3-methyl-2-butanone)-dioxime {PnAO}, labelled with $^{99m}$Tc. Fair *et al.*[19] characterized the complex with $^{99}$Tc and showed that the technetium core was formally $[Tc(V)O]^{3+}$. The PnAO ligand had reacted with the loss of three protons to give an overall neutral complex charge, $[Tc(V)OL]$. Complexation at the tracer level ($^{99m}$Tc) resulted in the formation of a neutral complex which when investigated in rats showed some brain uptake (1.3 per cent i.d. at 15 s p.i.) followed by rapid wash-out (0.036 per cent i.d. at 1 h p.i.).[67]

Several groups developed the diaminodithiol ($N_2S_2$) ligands. In all cases, the technetium complex formed was neutral, square pyramidal and based on a $[Tc(V)O]^{3+}$ core however, not all of these complexes exhibited the desired biological behaviour at the tracer level[4,36].

A neutral charge therefore is not the only prerequisite to brain uptake. Lipid solubility or octanol:water partition coefficients also have significant influence. The partition coefficient (P) is an indicator of lipophilicity (meaning fat-loving) and Dischino *et al.*[16] showed that there was a range of P values within which substrates will diffuse across the BBB. This range is accepted to be 0.9 < Log P>2.5. Morgan *et al.*[48] studied a series of ligands based on a custom-designed chelate which would neutralize a Tc(V)oxo core. The chelate structure allowed substitution into the ligand backbone which would have minimal effect on the co-ordinating atoms but would alter the lipophilic nature of the ligand and resulting technetium complex. Cerebral (and myocardial) uptake were noticeably altered and one of these ligands (MRP20) progressed to Phase II trials.

The molecular weight of the overall complex also plays a significant role. Levin[41] has reported that for transport across the BBB, the molecular weight should be under 400 Daltons. Neutral complexes with molecular weights in excess of 400 were more likely to be actively excreted by the liver.

An overall neutral complex charge and lipid solubility are required for passive diffusion of the technetium tracer across the BBB. Using elegant template complexation, the dioximes were developed by Narra *et al.*[52] as a separate class of compounds, the seven co-ordinated Tc(III) BATO complexes. The neutral Tc(III) dioximes were tested for both myocardial and cerebral perfusion. One of these, Tc(III)Cl(DMG)$_3$2MP was developed as a tracer for rCBF but not submitted for commercial approval. The complexes formed were very stable and there was no method of trapping the tracer within the brain, consequently, the tracer was excreted intact and wash-out occurred relatively quickly. A series of well-characterized neutral seven co-ordinate Tc(III) xanthate complexes were reported by Morgan *et al.*[49]. The xanthates are close congeners to the diethyldithiocarbamates (Fig. 4c) and in the presence of a neutral ligand such as triphenylphosphine P(Ph)$_3$ readily form stable, lipophilic complexes of the type [Tc(ligand)$_3$(PPh$_3$)]. Pre-clinical testing showed the versatility of this class of complex as both ligand and the neutral donor in the seventh co-ordinating position could be altered to optimize the biological results.

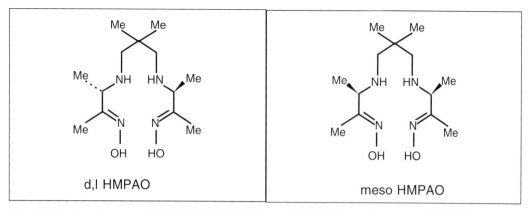

d,l HMPAO

meso HMPAO

*Fig. 6a Diastereoisomers of HMPAO: d,l HMPAO.*     *Fig. 6b Diastereoisomers of HMPAO: Meso HMPAO*

It was evident that for a radiopharmaceutical to be useful for brain SPET studies, a mechanism which trapped the tracer in the brain had to be designed into the ligand. Many derivatives of PnAO were synthesized and studied before the most appropriate chelating ligand was identified. This ligand was d,l-HMPAO (Fig. 6a), later commercialized as Ceretec™.

The ligand d,l-HMPAO is stable but when complexed with [$^{99m}$Tc]NaTcO$_4$ in saline solution in the presence of stannous ions, formed a neutral [Tc(V)OL] complex which possessed an inherent instability. Neirinckx *et al.*[53,54] showed that after intravenous injection of the radiopharmaceutical, the complex crossed the BBB with a first-pass extraction efficiency of 70–80 per cent and converted to a secondary more hydrophilic species which did not diffuse back out of the brain. The mechanism of fixation (or trapping) is thought to be a simple chemical interaction with glutathione, present as free thiol in millimolar concentration in the cells[61]. This theory has been supported by several *in vitro* studies but is not universally accepted and other parameters have been suggested, including protein binding in the cytosol[9]. Recently the role of glutathione was again questioned by Babich[1] but an alternative credible hypothesis has not been proffered.

The simultaneous development of the N$_2$S$_2$ ligands lead to the clinical testing of another series of compounds of which l,l-ethyl cysteinate dimer (ECD, Fig. 7a) has progressed to regulatory approval. $^{99m}$Tc-l,l-ECD is a neutral, lipid soluble Tc(V) complex which has been shown by Léveillé *et al.*[40] to be efficacious in humans. Following intravenous injection and passage across the BBB, two-step hydrolysis of the functional ester groups to carboxylic acids takes place. This results in an overall negative charge on the complex which prevents wash-out of the tracer from the brain tissue. The esterase responsible for the hydrolysis is as yet unidentified but is assumed to be ubiquitous throughout brain tissue[69].

The effect on biodistribution of the stereochemical arrangement of the chelating ligand is also known. The ligand HMPAO is synthesized as diastereoisomers. Sharp *et al.*[60] demonstrated in human volunteers that the per cent uptake in the brain of the technetium complex varies as a function of the stereoisomer. Tc-d,L-HMPAO shows superior brain uptake as compared to Tc-*meso*-HMPAO (Fig. 6b) and racemic mixtures of d,l- and *meso*-HMPAO result in an overall Tc-HMPAO complex that has significantly reduced brain uptake. Similarly, Walovitch[68] showed a significant difference in the hydrolysis of Tc-d,d-ECD (Fig. 7b) and Tc-l,l-ECD with the latter being the superior and preferred isomer. The enzyme responsible for the de-esterification of the complex appears to operate selectively on the Tc complex derived from the l,l isomer.

In the design of a suitable radiopharmaceutical, it is clear that delivery across the BBB is

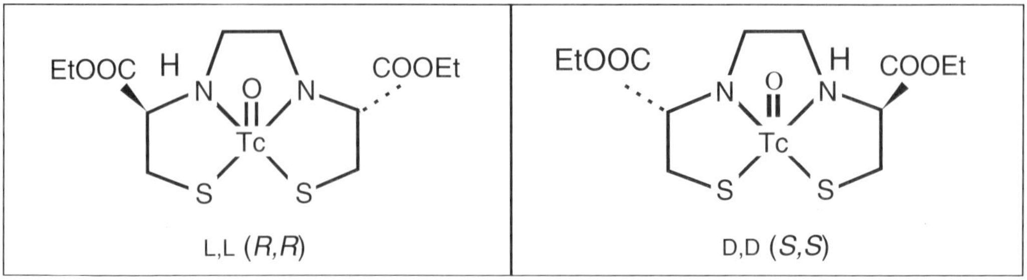

*Fig. 7a (left) and 7b (right) Tc-ECD stereoisomers.*

governed by simple physico-chemical characteristics. The 'art' of the science is to design a molecule which either possesses an inherent trapping mechanism or utilizes the natural chemical pathways available in the brain. Over the past decade, many different ligand classes have been investigated with the ultimate goal of producing the 'chemical microsphere' for cerebral perfusion imaging. If that ultimate goal implies qualitative and quantitative analysis of rCBF then it is not yet fully achieved. Methods for quantification of rCBF with $^{99m}$Tc-HMPAO have been reported but have not yet received wide acceptance as being useful in routine clinical practice and most routine clinical diagnoses with $^{99m}$Tc are made on qualitative and semi-quantitative analyses. The semi-quantitative analyses are becoming increasingly accurate as clinicians' experience with brain function increases. Absolute quantification is still achieved using $^{133}$Xe where the appropriate hardware is available and camera manufacturers are currently improving the acquisition algorithms for $^{133}$Xe to improve the resolution of the SPECT images. The availability of $^{127}$Xe would allow simultaneous imaging and quantitation to be performed but, to date, the production costs of $^{127}$Xe and the clinical management of an isotope with a $t_{1/2}$ of 36 days precludes its use in routine practice.

At the time of writing, one technetium cerebral perfusion tracer is commercially available, one is in advanced stages of regulatory approval and others are under clinical evaluation. Very recently the single-pass cerebral extraction and capillary permeability-surface area product of several of these brain perfusion tracers have been compared in rats using $^{85}$Strontium-labelled polystyrene microspheres to measure blood flow and $^{99m}$Tc-DTPA as control of the BBB permeability[15]. Interestingly, it is shown that at a cerebral blood flow level corresponding to normal regional CBF for human cortex, 0.5 ml/g/min, all the agents have a single-pass extraction of approximately 70 per cent or greater. All the agents detected CBF changes in the normal to ischaemic range. At higher flow rates $^{123}$I-IMP and $^{99m}$Tc-HMPAO demonstrated substantially greater fidelity to true CBF than $^{99m}$Tc-Cl(DMG)$_3$2MP and $^{99m}$Tc-ECD. Several other papers and review articles compare the technical and clinical characteristics of these tracers and the interested reader is referred to them.

Some clinical examples of perfusion studies with a $^{99m}$Tc-labelled tracer (Ceretec) and SPET are presented in the Appendix.

## References

1.  Babich, J. (1991): Technetium-99m-HMPAO retention and the role of glutathione: the debate continues. *J. Nucl. Med.* **32**, 1981–1983.

2.  Ballinger, J.R., Gerson, B. & Gulenchyn, K.Y. (1989): Technetium-99m dithiocarbamates as potential brain agents: evaluation of aliphatic and amine containing analogues. *Nucl. Med. Biol.* **16**, 721–725.

3.  Black, H.L., Hawkins, R.A., Kim, K.T., *et al.* (1989): Thallium-201 (SPECT): a quantitative technique to distinguish low grade from malignant brain tumours. *J. Neurosurg.* **71**, 342–346.

4.    Bok, B.D., Scheffel, U., Goldfarb, H.W., Burns, H.D., Lever, S.Z., Wong, D.F., Bice, A. & Wagner, H.N. Jr. (1987): Comparison of $^{99m}$Tc complexes (NEP-DADT, Me-NEP-DADT and HMPAO) with $^{123}$I-AMP for brain SPECT imaging in dogs. *Nucl. Med. Comm.* **8**, 631–641.

5.    Burke, J.W., Podrasky, A.E. & Bradley, W.G. (1990): Meninges: benign postoperative enhancement on MR images. *Radiology* **174**, 99–102.

6.    de Bruine, J.F., Van Royen, E.A., Vyth, A., de Jong, J.M.B.V. & Van der Schoot, J.B. (1985): Thallium-201 diethyldithiocarbamate: an alternative to iodine-123 *N*-isopropyl-*p*-iodo amphetamine. *J. Nucl. Med.* **26**, 925–930.

7.    Carrill, J.M., MacDonald, A.F., Dendy, P.P., Keyes, W.I., Umdnill, P.E. & Mallard, J.R. (1979): Cranial scintigraphy: value of adding emission computed tomography sections to conventional pertechnetate images (512 cases). *J. Nucl. Med.* **20**, 1117–1123.

8.    Carvalho, P.A., Schwartz, R.B., Alexander III, E., Loeffler, J. *et al.* (1991): Quantitative estimation of malignant glioma recurrence after radiotherapy. *J. Nucl. Med.* **32**, 933–939.

9.    Costa, D.C., Lui, D., Sinha, A.K., Jarritt, P.H. & Ell, P.J. (1989): Intracellular localisation of $^{99m}$Tc-d,l,-HMPAO and $^{201}$Tl-DDC in rat brain. *Nucl. Med. Comm.* **10**, 459–466.

10.   Dendy, P.P., McNab, J.W., MacDonald, A.F., Keyes, W.I. & Carrill, J.M. (1977): An evaluation of transverse axial emission tomography of the brain in the clinical situation. *Br. J. Radiol.* **50**, 555–561.

11.   Devous, M.D. Sr., Lowe, J.L. & Payne, J.K. (1992): Dual-isotope brain SPECT imaging with technetium-99m and Iodine-123: validation by phantom studies. *J. Nucl. Med.* **33(11)**, 2030–2035.

12.   Devous, M.D. Sr., Payne, J.K. & Lowe, J.L. (1992): Dual-isotope brain SPECT imaging with technetium-99m and iodine-123: clinical validation using xenon-133 SPECT. *J. Nucl. Med.* **33(11)**, 1919–1924.

13.   Di Chiro, G. (1986): Positron emission tomography using $^{18}$F-fluorodeoxyglucose in brain tumours: a powerful diagnostic and prognostic tool. *Invest. Radiol.* **22**, 360–371.

14.   Di Chiro, G. (1991): Which PET radiopharmaceutical for brain tumours? *J. Nucl. Med.* **32**, 1346–1348.

15.   Di Rocco, R.J., Silva, D.A., Kuczynski, B.L., Narra, R.K., Ramalingam, K., Jurisson, S., Nunn, A.D. & Eckelman, W.C. (1993): The single-pass cerebral extraction and capillary permeability-surface area product of several putative cerebral blood flow imaging agents. *J. Nucl. Med.* **34**, 641–648.

16.   Dischino, D.D., Welch, M.J., Kilbourm, M.R. & Raichle, M.E. (1983): Relationship between lipophilicity and brain extraction of $^{11}$C-labelled radiopharmaceuticals. *J. Nucl. Med.* **24**, 1030–1038.

17.   Ell, P.J., Deacon, J.M., Ducassou, D. & Brendel, A. (1980): Emission and transmission brain tomography. *Br. Med. J.* **280**, 438–440.

18.   Elster, A.D. & DiPersio, D.A. (1990): Cranial postoperative site: assessment with contrast-enhanced MR imaging. *Radiology* **174**, 93–98.

19.   Fair, C.K., Troutner, D.E., Schlemper, E.O., Murmann, R.K. & Hoppe, M.L. (1984): Oxo [3,3′-(1,3-propanediyldiimino)bis(3-methyl-2-butanone-oximato)(3-)*N*,*N*′,*N*′,*N*″] technetium (V), [TcO]Cl₃H₂₁₅N₄O₂) *Acta Cryst.* **C40**, 1544–1546.

20.   Gerlit, J.B. (1956): Some chemical properties of technetium. *Proc.Int.Conference Peaceful Uses of Atomic Energy* **7**, 145.

21.   Gibbs, J.M., Wise, R.J.S., Leenders, K. & Jones, T. (1984): Evaluation of perfusion reserve in patients with carotid artery occlusion. *Lancet* **i**, 310–314.

22.   Gibbs, J.M., Wise, R.J.S., Mansfield, A.O., Ross Russel, R., Thomas, D.J. & Jones, T. (1985): Regional cerebral blood flow and blood volume before and after EC–IC bypass surgery and carotid endarterectomy in patients with carotid artery disease. *J. Cereb. Blood Flow Metab.* **5** (suppl), 519–520.

23.   Glantz, M.J., Hoffman, J.M., Coleman, R.E., Friedman, A.H., Hanson, M.W., Burger, P.C., Herndon, J.E., Meisler, W.J. & Schold Jr, S.C. (1991): Identification of early recurrence of primary central nervous system tumours by [$^{18}$F]fluorodeoxyglucose positron emission tomography. *Ann. Neurol.* **29**, 347–355.

24.   Greenberg, J.H., Kushner, M., Rango, M., Alavi, A. & Reivich, M. (1990): Validation studies of Iodine-123-iodoamphetamine as a cerebral blood flow tracer using emission tomography. *J. Nucl. Med.* **31**, 1364–1369.

25.   Gruber, M.L. & Hochberg, F.H. (1990): Editorial: systematic evaluation of primary brain tumours. *J. Nucl. Med.* **31**, 969–971.

26.   Harper, P.V. (1965): Tc-99m as a scanning agent. *Radiology* **85**, 101.

27.    Hill, Th., Lovett, R.D. & McNeil, B.J. (1980): Observations on the clinical value of emission tomography. *J. Nucl. Med.* **21**, 613–616.

28.    Hoh, C.K., Khanna, S., Harris, G.C., Chen, T.T., Black, K.L., Becker, D.P., Maddahi, J., Marciano, D.M. & Hawkins, R.A. (1992): Evaluation of brain tumour recurrence with Thallium-201 SPECT studies: correlation with FDG PET and histological results. *J. Nucl. Med.* **33**, 867.

29.    Ingvar, D.H. & Lassen, N.A. (1961): Quantitative determination of regional cerebral blood flow in man. *Lancet* **ii**, 806–807.

30.    Kaplan, W.D., Takronan, T., Morris, H. *et al.* (1987): Thallium-201 brain tumour imaging: a comparative study with pathological correlation. *J. Nucl. Med.* **28**, 47–52.

31.    Kety, S.S. & Schmidt, C.F. (1948): Nitrous oxide method for the quantitative determination of cerebral blood flow in man: theory, procedure and normal values. *J. Clin. Invest.* **27**, 475–483.

32.    Kim, K.T., Black, K.L., Marciano, D. *et al.* (1990): Thallium-201 SPECT imaging of brain tumours: methods and results. *J. Nucl. Med.* **31**, 965–969.

33.    Knapp, W.H., Von Kummaer, R. & Kubler, W. (1986): Imaging of cerebral blood flow to volume distribution using SPECT. *J. Nucl. Med.* **27**, 465–470.

34.    Krishna, L., Slizofski, W.J., Katsetos, C.D., Nair, S., Dadparvar, S., Brown, S.J., Chevres, A. & Roman, R. (1992): Abnormal intracerebral thallium localization in a bacterial brain abscess. *J. Nucl. Med.* **33**, 2017–2019.

35.    Kuhl, D.E., Barrio, J.R., Huang, S.-C., Selin, C., Ackermann, R.F., Lear, J.L., Wu, J.L., Lin, T.N. & Phelps, M.E. (1982): Quantifying local cerebral blood flow by $N$-isopropyl-$p$-$^{123}$I-iodoamphetamine (IMP) tomography. *J. Nucl. Med.* **2**, 196–203

36.    Kung, H.F. & Blau, M. (1980): Regional intracellular pH shift: a proposed new mechanism for radiopharmaceutical uptake in brain and other tissues. *J. Nucl. Med.* **21**, 147–152.

37.    Kung, H.F., Guo, Y.Z., Yu Chi-Chou, Billings, J., Subramanyam, V. & Calabrese J.C. (1989): New brain perfusion imaging agents based on $^{99m}$Tc-bis(aminoethanethiol) complexes: stereoisomers and biodistribution. *J. Med. Chem.* **32**, 433–437.

38.    Lear, J.L. & Navarro, D. (1987): Autoradiographic comparison of Thallium-201 diethyldithiocarbamate, isopropyliodoamphetamine and iodoantipyrine as cerebral blood flow tracers. *J. Nucl. Med.* **28**, 481–486.

39.    Lebowitz, E., Greene, M.W., Fairchild, R., Bradley-Moore, P.R., Atkins, H.L., Ansari, A.N., Richards, P. & Belgrave, E. (1975): Thallium-201 for medical use, I. *J. Nucl. Med.* **16**, 151–160.

40.    Léveillé, J., Demonceau, G., De Roo, M., Rigo, P., Taillefer, R., Morgan, R.A., Kupranick, D. & Walovitch, R.C. (1989): Characterisation of Tc-99m-L,L-ECD for brain perfusion imaging, Part 2: Biodistribution and brain imaging in humans. *J. Nucl. Med.* **30**, 1902–1910.

41.    Levin, V.A. (1980): Relationship of octanol/water partition coefficient and molecular weight to rat brain capillary permeability. *J. Med. Chem.* **23**, 682–684.

42.    Loberg, M.D., Corder, E.H., Fields, A.T. & Callery, P.S. (1979): Membrane transport of $^{99m}$Tc-labelled radiopharmaceuticals. 1. Brain uptake by passive transport. *J. Nucl. Med.* **20(11)**, 1181–1188.

43.    Loeffler, J.S., Siddon, R.L., Wen, P.Y., Nedzi, L.A. & Alexander, E.A. III (1989): Stereotactic radiosurgery of the brain using a standard linear accelerator: a study of early and late effects. *Radiother. Oncol.* **17**, 311–321.

44.    Loken, M.K. (1985): A history of clinical nuclear medicine. In: *Nuclear medicine annual*, eds. L.M. Freeman & H.S. Weissmann, pp. 1–21. New York: Raven Press.

45.    Maier-Hauff, K., Barzen, G.S. & Gottschalk, H. (1992): Value of $^{201}$Tl imaging in cerebral lesions: emission CT with autoradiography. *Radiology* **185(P)**, 232–2332.

46.    Moore, G.E. (1947): Fluorescin as an agent in the differentiation of normal and malignant tissues. *Science, NY* **106**, 130–131.

47.    Moore, G.E. (1948): The use of radioactive diiodofluorescin in the diagnosis and localization of brain tumours. *Science, NY* **107**, 569.

48.    Morgan, G.F., Abram, U., Evrard, G., Durant, F., Deblaton, M., Clemens, P., Van den Broeck, P. & Thornback, J.R. (1990): Structural characterisation of the new brain imaging agent, $[^{99m}$Tc][TcO(L)], H₃L = $N$-4-oxopentan-2-ylidene-$N'$-pyrrol-2-ylmethylethane-1,2-diamine. *J. Chem. Soc. Chem. Commun.* 1772–1773.

49. Morgan, G.F., Thornback, J.R., Delmon, L., Jones, A.G., Nicholson, T. & Davison, A. (1990): Seven coordinate technetium xanthate complexes: a novel class of compounds with potential in nuclear medicine. In: *Nuclear-medizine. Quantitative analysis in imaging and function*, eds. H.A.E. Schmidt and J. Chambron, pp. 84–86. Stuttgart: Schattauer.

50. Mori, H., Shiba, K., Matsuda, H., Tsuji, S. & Hisada, K. (1990): Characteristics of the binding of *N*-isopropyl-*p*-[125]I-iodoamphetamine in the rat brain synaptosomal membranes. *Nucl. Med. Comm.* **11**, 327–331.

51. Mosskin, M., Von Holst, H., Bergstrom, M., Collins, V.P., Erikson, L., Johnstrom, P. & Noren, G. (1987): Positron emission tomography with [11]C-methionine and computed tomography of intracranial tumours compared with histopathologic examination of multiple biopsies. *Acta Radiol.* **28**, 505–509.

52. Narra, R.K., Nunn, A.D., Kuczynski, B.L., Di Rocco, R.J., Feld, T., Silva, D.A. & Eckelman, W.C. (1990): A neutral lipophilic Technetium-99m complex for regional cerebral blood flow imaging. *J. Nucl. Med.* **31** 1370–1377.

53. Neirinckx, R.D., Canning, L.R., Piper, I.M., Nowotnik, D.P., Pickett, R.D., Holmes, R.A., Volkert, W.A., Forster, A.M., Weisner, P.S., Marriott, J.A. & Chaplin, S.B. (1987): Tc-99m-d,l-HMPAO: a new radiopharmaceutical for SPECT imaging of regional cerebral blood perfusion. *J. Nucl. Med.* **28**, 191–202.

54. Neirinckx, R.D., Nowotnik, D.P., Pickett, R.D., Harrison, R.C. & Ell, P.J. (1986): Development of a lipophilic [99m]Tc complex useful for brain perfusion evaluation with conventional SPECT imaging equipment. In: *Amphetamines and pH shift agents for brain imaging. Basic research and clinical results*, eds, H.J. Biersack & C. Winkler, pp. 59–70. Berlin: Walter de Gruyter.

55. Reivich, M., Kuhl, D., Wolf, A. *et al.* (1979): The [18]F-fluorodeoxyglucose method for the measurement of local cerebral glucose utilisation in man. *Circ. Res.* **44**, 127–137.

56. Rossman, D.J., Strauss, H.W., Siegel, M.E. *et al.* (1975): Accumulation of [99m]Tc-glucoheptonate in acutely infarcted myocardium. *J. Nucl. Med.* **16**, 875–878.

57. Ryerson, T.W., Spies, S.M., Singh, N.B. & Zeman, R.K. (1978): A quantitative clinical comparison of three [99m]Tc-labelled brain imaging radiopharmaceuticals. *Radiology* **127**, 429–432.

58. Rollo, F.D., Cavalieri, R.R., Born, M., Blei, L. & Chew, M. (1977): Comparative evaluation of [99m]Tc-GH, [99m]TcO4, and [99m]Tc-DTPA as brain imaging agents. *Radiology* **123**, 379–383.

59. Schwartz, R.B., Carvalho, P.A., Alexander III, E., Loeffler, J.S., Folkerth, R. & Holman, B.L. (1992): Radiation necrosis *vs* high-grade recurrent glioma: differentiation by using dual-isotope SPECT with [201]Tl and [99m]Tc-HMPAO. *Am. J. Neuro. Radiol.* **12**, 1187–1192.

60. Sharp, P.F., Smith, F.W., Gemmell, H.G., Lyall, D., Evans, N.T.S., Gvozdanovic, D., Davison, J., Dyrell, D.A., Pickett, R.D. & Neirinckx, R.D. (1986): Tc-99m HMPAO stereoisomers as potential agents for imaging regional cerebral blood flow: human volunteer studies. *J. Nucl. Med.* **27**, 171–177.

61. Suess, E., Malessa, S., Ungersböck, K., Kitz, P., Podreka, I., Heimberger, K., Hornykiewicz, O. & Deeke, L. (1991): Tc-99m-d,l-Hexamethylpropyleneamine Oxime (HMPAO) uptake and glutathione content in brain tumours. *J. Nucl. Med.*. **32(9)**, 1675–1681.

62. Takeshita, G., Maeda, H., Nakane, K., Toyama, H., Sakakibara, E., Komai, S., Takenchi, A., Koga, S., Ono, M. & Nakagawa, T. (1992): Quantitative measurements of regional cerebral blood flow using *N*-isopropyl-(iodine-123)*p*-iodoamphetamine and single photon emission computed tomography. *J. Nucl. Med.* **33**, 1741–1749.

63. Troutner, D.E., Volkert, W.A., Hoffman, T.J. & Holmes, R.A. (1984): A neutral lipophilic complex of [99m]Tc with a multidentate amine oxime. *Int. J. Appl. Radiat. Isot.* **35**, 467–470.

64. Uszler, J.M., Bennett, L.R., Mena, I. & Oldendorf, W.H. (1975): Human CNS perfusion scanning with [123]I-iodoantipyrine. *Radiology* **115**, 197–200.

65. Valk, P.E., Budinger, T.F., Levin, V.A., Silver, P., Cutin, P.H. & Doyle, W.K. (1988): PET of malignant cerebral tumours after interstitial brachytherapy: demonstration of metabolic activity and correlation with clinical outcome. *J. Neurosurg.*, **69**, 830–838.

66. Van Royen, E.A. (1987): Thallium-201 DDC: an alternative radiopharmaceutical for rCBF. *Nucl. Med. Commun.* **8**, 603–610.

67. Volkert, W.A., McKenzie, E.H., Hoffman, T.J., Troutner, D.E. & Holmes, R.A. (1984): The behaviour of neutral amine oxime chelates labelled with Tc at tracer level. *Int. J. Nucl. Med. Biol.* **11**, 243–246.

68. Walovitch, R.C., Franceschi, M., Picard, M., Cheesman, E.H., Hall, K.M., Makuch, J., Watson, M.W., Zimmerman, R.E., Watson, A.D., Ganey, M.V., Williams, S.J. & Holman, B.L. (1991): Metabolism of [99m]Tc-L,L-Ethyl cysteinate dimer in healthy volunteers. *Neuropharmacology* **30**, 283–292.

69.     Walovitch, R.C., Hill, T.C., Garrity, S.T., Cheesman, E.H., Burgess, B.A., O'Leary, D.H., Watson, A.D., Ganey, M.V., Morgan, R.A. & Williams, S.J. (1989): Characterisation of Tc-99m-L,L-ECD for brain perfusion imaging, part 1: pharmacology of Tc-99m ECD in nonhuman primates. *J. Nucl. Med.* **30**, 1892–1901.

70.     Warburg, O. (1930): *The metabolism of tumours*, pp. 75–?327. London: Arnold Constable.

71.     Watson, N.E., Cowan, R.J., Ball, M.R., Moody, D.M., Lastee, D.W. & Maynard, C.D. (1980): A comparison of brain imaging with gamma camera, single photon emission computed tomography and transmission computed tomography. *J. Nucl. Med.* **21**, 507–511.

72.     Waxman, A.D., Tanacescu, D., Siemsen, J.K. & Wolfstein, R.S. (1976): Tc-99m-glucoheptonate as a brain scanning agent: critical comparison with pertechnetate. *J. Nucl. Med.* **17**, 345–348.

73.     Winchell, H.S., Baldwin, R.M. & Lin, T.H. (1980): Development of [123]I-labelled amines for brain studies: localisation of I-123 iodophenylalkyl amines in rat brain. *J. Nucl. Med.* **21**, 940–946.

74.     Zweiman, F.G., O'Keefe, A., Idoine J. *et al.* (1974): Selective uptake of [99m]Tc chelates and [67]Ga in acutely infarcted myocardium. *J. Nucl. Med.* **15**, 546–547.

## Further reading

Cowan, R.J. (1986): Conventional radionuclide brain imaging in the era of transmission and emission tomography. *Sem. Nucl. Med.* **XVI**, 63–73.

Early, P.J. and Sodee, D.B. (1985): *Principles and practice of nuclear medicine*. St. Louis, Toronto: C.V. Mosby

Saha, G.B. (1984): *Fundamentals of nuclear pharmacy*, 2nd edition. New York: Springer.

*New Trends in Nuclear Neurology and Psychiatry*, edited by D.C. Costa, G.F. Morgan and N. A. Lassen
© 1993 John Libbey & Company Ltd., pp. 85–100

# Chapter 6

## Studying *in vivo* brain chemistry with SPECT: receptors and neurotransmission

B. Mazière and M. Mazière

*Service Hospitalier Frédéric Joliot, Direction des Sciences du Vivant, Commissariat à l'Energie Atomique, 91406 Orsay, France*

### Introduction

During the 1960s, brain radioisotopic imaging knew its first success in the domain of anatomic imaging using planar scintigraphy and radiopharmaceuticals such as pertechnetate or DTPA-labelled with $^{99m}$Tc that permitted the study of blood–brain barrier modifications linked to tumours, abscess or strokes. Subsequently, the first 'functional' images of the brain were obtained with the visualization of cerebral blood volume using proteins or red cells labelled with $^{99m}$Tc or $^{111}$In.

Functional imaging developed considerably during the 1970s with the simultaneous use of positron emission tomography (PET) and specific radiopharmaceuticals. Recent progress in our understanding of the mechanisms involved in neurotransmission processes is mainly due to the technical revolutions that have arisen, in the field of neuroscience, during the last decade. Amongst them, emission tomography visualization techniques, such as PET and single photon emission computerized tomography (SPECT), have offered new possibilities in clinical investigation for the *in vivo* study of the physiology and the pathology of the human brain and heart. The measurement of regional biochemical functions requires the use of endogenous or exogenous labelled molecules that participate in a given metabolic process. Thus the design of a tracer is based on physiological concepts such as metabolic turnover (oxygen, glucose, amino acids, fatty acids), immuno-reaction, enzyme concentration or activity, neurotransmitter biochemistry, receptor occupancy or density. Using such specific radiotracers labelled with positron or gamma-emitting radioisotopes and gamma-ray detection systems (positron camera or rotating gamma-camera) for external detection, it is now possible to measure, in an atraumatic way, local tissue functions (glucose and oxygen utilization), pH, cerebral blood flow and neurotransmission systems (receptors-neurotransmitters).

PET and SPECT each have their inherent advantages and drawbacks: for PET, general problems of attenuation (independent of the position of the radioactive source inside the body, and scatter corrections (inherent directionality of the pair of photons accompanying positron annihilation) have been reasonably resolved and absolute radionuclide quantitation *in situ* is now routine. On the contrary, for SPECT, accurate, generally applicable corrections for attenuation and scatter are not yet routinely available. The low sensitivity of rotating scintillation camera-based SPECT is also a major limitation: the current sensitivity of a SPECT device is typically one to two orders of magnitude lower than that of PET. However, the wider availability of SPET instrumentation is an advantage over PET when studying large population samples. In addition, dedicated brain imaging systems and the introduction of better algorithms for attenuation correction (transmission/emission tomography – see Chapter 4) will further favour the use of SPET. The problem lies in the development of new radiotracers as the chemistry of technetium and iodine is more complex than that related to $^{11}$C and $^{15}$O labelling.

At the turn of the century, Langley[52] formulated the concept of 'receptive substances' involved in the origin of the pharmacological response to drugs. This idea was quickly extended to explain most of the modes of action of substances affecting the nerve terminals and the term 'receptor' was soon coined by Erhlich (1910). Several decades later, the extensive use of tritiated ligands having high specific radioactivities (curies per millimole), allowed the *in vitro* measurement of minute concentrations of brain neuroreceptors (ca. $10^{-12}$ mole per gram), their biochemical characterization (using 'binding' techniques) and their visualization (using *in vitro* or *in vivo* autoradiography). By substituting positron emitting or medium or high energy gamma-ray emitting radioisotopes for tritium and by using an appropriate external imaging device (positron or rotating gamma camera) it was possible to obtain, in a living subject, an accurate representation of the spatial distribution of a gamma-emitting radionuclide[38] and then the quantitative image of the distribution of a previously administered radiolabelled ligand.

The tomographic approach for receptor study is analogous to that used in quantitative auto radiography. Moreover, whichever technique is used (PET or SPECT) emission tomography allows *in vivo* sequential studies. The serial images obtained give the opportunity to calculate, in selected regions of interest, activity versus time curves. Tomographic methods are safe and non invasive due to the short half-life of the radioisotopes used. Radiation dosimetry to organs of the human body following administration of radioligands labelled with $^{123}$I have shown acceptable estimates for effective dose equivalents (EDE). An example is given by the study undertaken by Thonoor *et al.* [96] with an iodinated dopamine $D_1$ receptor imaging agent which showed that, for the dose usually injected (3–5 mCi for $^{123}$I-ligands), the resultant radiation dose absorbed by the critical target organs i.e. liver, lower larger intestine, bladder) remained within the accepted 5 rad per organ limit per single study.

All *in vivo* techniques studying brain functions including the tomographic approach have limitations as different serial physiological barriers are present between the site of administration (a brachial vein in humans) and the brain tissue itself. The first barrier is the pulmonary filter : In a single passage through the lung circulation, lipophilic molecules can be totally extracted by the pulmonary endothelial or epithelial cells; in such conditions, the amount of ligand that will reach the receptors will depend on its clearance from the lungs. The second barrier is the capillary barrier and this problem is very acute in the brain where the intercellular junctions are very tight, the permeability of the BBB being higher for molecules that enter the lipid matrix of the endothelial cell membrane more readily. Another obstacle to the brain uptake of tracers is the binding of the labelled molecule to plasma proteins, the degree of which is independent of its lipophilicity.

**Receptor binding studies**

The best approach when labelling a pharmacologically active molecule for external detection is the replacement of one of its original atoms by a gamma-emitting isotope. When such an isotopic

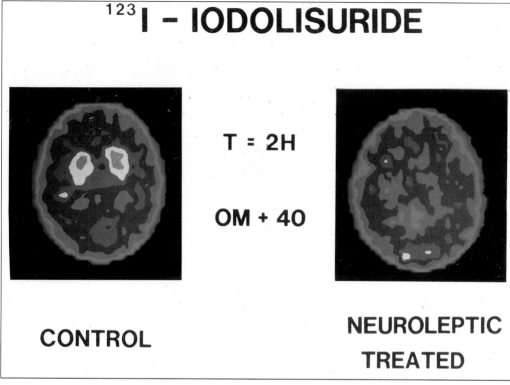

*Fig. 1. Tomographic images obtained 2 h after intravenous administration of 5 mCi of the dopamine re-ceptor antagonist iodolisuride labelled with [123]I in a control subject (left) and in a schizophrenic pa-tient treated with high doses of haloperidol (right).*

labelling is inconvenient, another approach can be considered: preparing a radiohalogenated analogue of the compound.

There is an enormous increase in the number of labelled ligands that have been prepared and evaluated for brain receptor mapping[64]. This is not only true for PET but also the number of [123]I-labelled ligands for SPECT is increasing.

One complication of tomographic receptor studies is related to the non-specific binding of the ligand (the lower the lipophilicity, the higher the specific to non-specific ratio) and its removal process within the tissue (uptake by different cells, binding to different receptors or different receptor subtypes, enzymatic or chemical degradation, intracellular trapping).

The binding of a ligand with a receptor exhibits two unique properties, molecular specificity and saturability, which will be used, *in vivo*, for receptor characterization. Molecular specificity describes the behaviour of ligand binding in terms of affinity and ability to recognize a particular molecule while saturability is related to receptor density. Brain tissue contains a minute concentration of receptors (approximately $10^{-12}$ mole per gram) and if a ligand is delivered in excess, the receptors will become saturated. Very low concentration of ligands must therefore be injected which implies the preparation of radioligands labelled at very high specific activities (above 18.5 MBq/nmol 0.5 mCi/nmol).

Thus there are several premises that have to be fulfilled for a ligand to be useful for SPECT (or PET) investigations:

- adequate lipophilicity for reasonable uptake in the brain and low non-specific binding;
- high specific / non-specific binding ratio;
- high affinity ($K_d$ nM) and selectivity;
- good metabolic stability during the time of experiment.

For sensitivity reasons, labelled endogenous neurotransmitters cannot be used for receptor mapping because of the high *in vivo* dilution with competing inactive ligands. Therefore, exogenous antagonists (or agonists) with high affinity and selectivity are exclusively used. The increasing receptor heterogeneity, due to advances in molecular pharmacology and biology has prompted the development of new subtype receptor ligands.

## Neurotransmission systems

Methods for the investigation of brain functions by PET have been available for several years; the study by PET of neuroreceptor characteristics in the living human brain was successfully demonstrated some years ago, and now applications in neurology, psychiatry and clinical psychopharmacology are currently published in the literature. Conversely, although SPECT has been available for 10 years, the method is still at a very early stage of application in receptor-binding problems. Successful PET tracers have the design and synthesis of corresponding [123]I analogues for SPECT investigations and potential brain receptor imaging agents labelled with [123]I are currently reported but largely their clinical potential for measuring changes in receptor-binding remains to be investigated.

## Dopaminergic system

The dopaminergic system is the first system in which it has been possible to image, using PET or SPECT, various pre- and post-synaptic steps of the chemical neurotransmission including receptors, stored neurotransmitter and neurotransmitter re-uptake mechanisms.

## Neurotransmitter regional metabolism

For SPECT investigation purposes, the radio-iodinated analogue of 6-fluoro-L-dopa, 6-[123]I-L-dopa, has been prepared[1]. Preliminary biodistribution results in rodents have suggested that the ratio striatum-to-whole brain is 1.35 (compared to 1.55 for 6-F-dopa). However, the low brain uptake observed in rats, if also apparent in man, would preclude its use for SPECT studies.

## Dopamine regulatory systems

Dopamine concentration in a synapse is partly regulated through pre-synaptic reuptake and enzymatic degradation by the monoamine oxydase enzymes.

Very recently, several ligands have been proposed to visualize dopamine reuptake sites using SPECT.

Preliminary studies on analogues of the dopamine uptake inhibitor GBR 12 935 have shown that ([123]I)-iodo-GBR could be a potential tool to explore the presynaptic step of the dopaminergic neurotransmission[25].

There is evidence that the powerful properties of cocaine stem from its inhibition of dopamine uptake. Of the three isomers of iodococaine which were prepared, the *para*-iodinated compound exhibited both the most and the greatest potency to displace tritiated cocaine from striatal membranes[71]. Carrier-free radio-iodinated cocaine imaging of the dog and baboon brain was recently reported[2,105]. Although rapid accumulation of activity in the brain and prolonged striatal clearance were observed, assessment of specific binding sites was not possible.

Several analogues of cocaine of the WIN series (the ester linkage of the benzoyl function has been eliminated) have been used previously as ligands for the dopamine reuptake site[8]. Of these, RTI-55 (also named CIT) has proven to be the most potent ligand.[123]I-RTI-55 has been prepared and evaluated in baboons[74]. The tracer exhibits SPECT uptake kinetics that reaches a pseudo-plateau after about 60 min and displays high specific binding in the striatum and hypothalamus, displaceable with citalopram (an agent selective for the serotonin reuptake site) and indatraline (a potent agent for the dopamine and serotonin reuptake sites). These *in vivo* SPECT displacement experiments support the notion that most of the striatal binding is associated with dopamine reuptake sites while the hypothalamic activity is associated with serotonin reuptake sites.

Twenty-four hours after intravenous administration of [123]I-RTI-55 in a baboon, the striatal to cerebellar ratio of radioactivity reached a value of 12. When the same study was performed in a MPTP-pretreated baboon, no radio tracer accumulation was observed in the striatum. [123]I-RTI-55 appears then to be a potential tracer for the clinical imaging of monoamine reuptake sites[34] including dopamine[89] and serotonin[82] reuptake sites.

A reversible inhibitor of[57] monoamine oxidase B (Ro 43-0463), labelled with [123]I and an iodinated analogue of the suicide inhibitor of monoamine oxidase A (clorgyline)[75] have shown either inhibitory potency or favourable distribution in rats and are presently considered for advanced developments.

## Dopamine receptors

Most scientists endorse the hypothesis that there are at least two major dopamine receptor types belonging to the G-protein-coupled family of receptor proteins. $D_1$ receptors are linked to the stimulation of adenylate cyclase and $D_2$ receptors are linked to the inhibition of this enzyme[42,91, 92]. These receptor subtypes mediate opposite effects in the central nervous system: $D_1$ receptors open while $D_2$ receptors close potassium channels resulting respectively in hyper-polarization and depolarization of the postsynaptic neurone[7]. $D_1$ receptors are thought to be located on intrinsic neurons within the corpus striatum whereas $D_2$ receptors exist mainly on axons and terminals of cortico-striatal pathways. Within the past two years, molecular genetic studies have revealed the existence of three further receptors of the same family: the $D_3$ and $D_4$ subtypes that resemble $D_2$, and the $D_5$ subtype that resembles more closely the $D_1$ subtype.

$D_1$ and $D_2$ receptors display separate and distinct functions in both physiology and in biochemistry[11]; however, the systemic administration of agonists for both subtypes produces synergistic effects on several behavioural responses and eventually induces akathisia in humans[24]. The ability to image $D_1$ and $D_2$ receptors could then be enlightening in the study of various movement disorders.

## D₁ dopamine receptors

To provide a PET localization of $D_1$ receptor in the living brain, benzazepine derivatives have been labelled with iso- or hetero-positron emitters.

To provide a SPECT localization of $D_1$ receptors, radio-iodinated analogues of the reference benzazepine compound, SCH 23390, have been prepared. According to the position of the radioactive iodine atom, these analogues have been named SCH 23982 or IBZP[4,48,66,90], FISCH[5,18] or TISCH[6]. *In vitro* and *in vivo* experiments in rats have shown that, compared to the original antagonist, these [125]I-radiolabelled analogues possess similar affinity and selectivity for the D1 receptor. In a preliminary experiment on a monkey, $^{123}$I-SCH 23982 was shown to accumulate in the basal ganglia[48] but the low striatum/cortex and striatum/cerebellum ratios combined with the short biological half-life of these compounds [$t_{1/2}$ < h] were a barrier to their utilization as SPECT clinical imaging agents. In contrast, the (+) isomer of ($^{123}$I)-TISCH showed high uptake in the basal ganglia and a relatively prolonged retention in the baboon[6]. The low radiation burden[72] estimated in healthy subjects with the absorbed fraction technique made it feasible to use this ligand for the non-invasive imaging of $D_1$ receptor in neuropsychiatric patients.

## D$_2$ dopamine receptors

It is generally assumed that the antipsychotic (but also the extra-pyramidal) effects of neuroleptics are mediated by a blockade of $D_2$ receptors since there is a strong correlation between the antipsychotic potency of these drugs and their *in vitro* affinity. So research on $D_2$ dopamine receptors could be considerably developed due to the availability of several selective antagonists belonging to the neuroleptic pharmacological family.

The agents of this family can be divided into different groups according to their chemical structures, namely phenothiazines, thioxantines, butyrophenones, diphenyl-piperidines, dibenzo-diazepines, benzamides and ergolenes. PET and SPECT investigations have been successfully undertaken with three of them: the radiolabelled butyrophenone, benzamide and ergolene derivatives.

For SPECT purposes, the *butyrophenone* spiperone has been labelled with $^{123}$I in two positions: either in the tertiary amine[67] or in the *p*-fluorobutyrophenone[78] moiety. The variable individual pharmacokinetics (in particular the affinity for $D_2$ dopamine receptors) and species dependency significantly influences their possible clinical utility. Despite a reasonable affinity of $^{123}$I-(4-iodo)spiperone for dopamine receptors, the high non-specific binding of this ligand does not offer useful prospects for SPECT clinical receptor imaging[99]. Better perspectives are probably offered by $^{123}$I-(2'-iodo)spiperone, encouraging results having been reported in preliminary baboon and human brain SPECT investigations[68,79]. Considering the interesting results obtained with the *N*-alkyl derivatives of spiperone labelled with $^{18}$F, $^{123}$I-iodinated *N*-alkyl[15,80] and *N*-allyl[53] spiperone analogues have also been prepared and have shown a potential for use in clinical studies.

However it is well known that spiperone and its derivatives also have a high affinity *in vivo* for central serotonin receptors[26]. Research on the development of more specific $D_2$ ligands have shown the value of other series of dopamine antagonists. Thus, the benzamide and the ergolene analogues, compared to spiperone derivatives, appear to be advantageous with regard to selectivity, rapidity of association and reversibility of specific binding.

Several radio iodinated *benzamides*, such as iodopride[38], iodosulpiride[59], IMB[102], spectramide[81], IBF[50], IBZM[49], iodotropapride[13], epidepride[40] and NCQ298[30], have been reported to show, *in vitro* and *in vivo* in animals, very high affinity and selectivity to the $D_2$ dopamine receptor.

For SPECT investigations, a radio-iodinated analogue of raclopride, $^{123}$I-IBZM, has been prepared and extensively studied. *Ex vivo* and *in vivo* images in rats and in a monkey demonstrated a high concentration in basal ganglia[49]. Unilateral denervation of the nigrostriatal dopamine system in primates and rodents has been shown to induce an increase in $^{123}$I-IBZM striatal binding that corresponded to dopamine agonist-induced behaviour[15,17].

*In vivo* amphetamine-stimulated dopamine release experiments in non-human primates have indicated that endogenous dopamine may effectively compete for $^{123}$I-IBZM striatal binding[37].

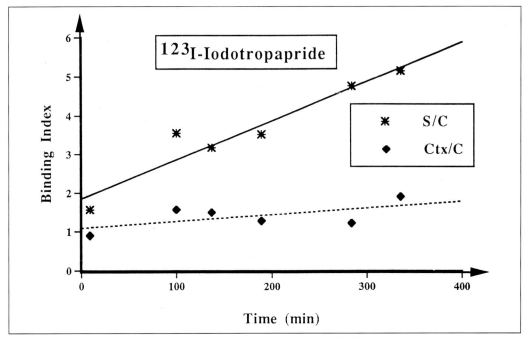

*Fig. 2. Time course of the binding indices striatum to cerebellum (S/C) and temporal cortex to cerebellum radioactive concentration ratio registered, with a single head rotating gamma camera, in a control subject injected with 5 mCi of [123]I-iodotropapride, a dopamine D₂ receptor antagonist.*

Serial [123]I-IBZM dynamic SPECT images acquired every 2 min and arterial blood measurements of unchanged radiopharmaceutical concentrations were used to assess[88] dynamic aspects of the uptake and wash-out of [123]I-IBZM brain activity.

In preliminary clinical SPECT investigations, [123]I-IBZM striatal fixation was markedly reduced in a patient on neuroleptic treatment[19]. [123]I-IBZM was then used to try to correlate central D2 dopamine receptor availability and clinical efficacy in schizophrenics treated with typical and atypical antipsychotic drugs[27,76]. In patients with chorea[12] and with neurological symptoms of Wilson's disease, [123]I-IBZM fixation in striata was markedly reduced[86,95]. In a prospective study, IBZM-SPECT was able to predict the response to dopamimetic therapy in patients with *de novo* parkinsonism[87].

Preliminary studies of radiohalogeno derivatives of tropapride in rats and baboons have demonstrated the potential of using nortropane-substituted benzamides to evaluate the status of central nervous system dopamine D2 receptors. In humans, [123]I-iodotropapride displays a slow accumulation in the striata; 4 h post injection, the specific binding index (striatum to cerebellum radioactive concentration ratio) measured with a single head rotating gamma camera was approximately 4 (Fig. 2)[56].

Epidepride, the iodine analogue of isoremoxipride (FLB457), was also found to be (with a $K_d$ of about 30 pM) a very potent dopamine D₂ receptor antagonist[40]. *In vivo*, rat brain uptake revealed a very high striatum to cerebellum ratio and a hippocampal/cerebellar and frontal cortical/cerebellar ratio of 2.2, reversible with a haloperidol pretreatment[43]. A preliminary SPECT study performed on a normal volunteer demonstrated that [123]I-epidepride can be successfully used to delineate extrastriatal dopamine $D_2$ receptors (in the thalamus, temporal lobe and hypothalamus and pituitary) in man[44].

NCQ298, the iodinated analogue benzamide of FLB463, was labelled with [123]I and studied in baboons with SPECT. The measured striatum to cerebellum ratio was about 15 at 3 h p.i.[30].

Among the *ergolenes*, the 2-halogeno derivatives of lisuride (2-bromo or 2-iodo lisuride) possess definite antidopaminergic properties. After labelling with [123]I, idolisuride (ILIS) has shown, in *in vivo* and *in vitro* animal experiments, identical affinity and selectivity to those of [76]Br-bromolisuride for $D_2$ receptors. Tomographic images, obtained in human controls using either a dedicated SPECT device or a rotating gamma-camera, have revealed an accumulation of the radioligand in the striatal structures (Fig. 1). This specific fixation, which disappeared in patients treated with high doses of haloperidol[55], was significantly reduced in patients with clinical evidence of progressive nuclear palsy[14,63] and increased in young girls with Rett syndrome[16].

## Serotoninergic system

### Serotonin uptake sites

The pharmacological action of many antidepressants, such as fluoxetine or imipramine are based on blockage of presynaptic reuptake sites for serotonin (or norepinephrine). Recently, imipramine[33], paroxetine[60], nitroquipazine[61] and tomoxetine[51] have been labelled with [125]I and used to characterize the serotonin reuptake site in rodents with varying degrees of success *in vitro* and *in vivo*.

The carbomethoxy phenyl tropane derivative, RTI-55, which in the brain binds *in vivo* to the reuptake sites of monoamines (including dopamine[89] and serotonin[74,82]), holds promise as a SPECT imaging agent for imaging serotonin transport in humans.

### Serotonin receptors

At least five receptor subtypes have been identified but *in vivo* specific radioligands have only been described for the $S_2$ and eventually the $S_1$ receptors.

In an attempt to develop a specific agent for $S_1$ brain imaging with SPECT, the potent serotonin agonist 8-hydroxy-PAT has been labelled with radioiodine. Despite a very high non-specific binding, the *in vivo* autoradiographs of rat brain have shown distribution patterns similar to those obtained with the tritiated ligand[47].

Various more or less selective $S_2$ agonists (DOI[65]) or antagonists (LSD[23], N-ethyl-LSD[54], ketanserin[69,70], amino-ketanserin[84]) have been labelled with radioiodine. Preliminary [123]I-ketanserin SPECT imaging studies have shown, in humans, distribution patterns corresponding to those found in post-mortem binding studies with [3]H-ketanserin. In baboons a frontal cortex to cerebellum ratio of 10 was achieved after 2 h. However this selective cortical binding could be inhibited by preloading the animal with cold ketanserin[9].

## Cholinergic System

### Cholinergic presynaptic markers: vesamicol receptors

Vesamicol, (–)*trans*-2-(4-phenylpiperidino)cyclohexanol, has been shown to bind in a stereoselective, non-competitive manner to a membrane component of acetylcholine-containing presynaptic vesicles at a site distinct from the transporter active site and to inhibit the presynaptic storage of acetylcholine. Autoradiographic studies have shown that vesamicol binding sites are highly localized on cholinergic nerve terminal regions. Vesamicol derivatives and analogues

(HIPP) have been recently labelled with [11]C[45], [18]F[101], and [125]I [22,41] and evaluated *ex vivo* and *in vivo* as SPECT and PET tracers. The preliminary results are encouraging and support the concept that these radiolabelled derivatives can be successfully used to image the distribution of vesamicol binding sites and thus presynaptic cholinergic neurones.

### *Cholinergic postsynaptic markers*

At the beginning of the century, acetylcholine receptors were subdivided into two main classes, nicotinic and muscarinic. Though nicotine blocks nicotinic receptors following an initial stimulation, it remains the reference agonist, whereas d-tubocurarine specifically antagonizes these nicotinic receptors. Up to now, no ligand labelled with [123]I has been described for this receptor subtype. For the muscarinic receptors, the reference agonist and antagonist respectively remains muscarine and atropine.

For SPECT investigations of the muscarinic receptors, QNB[21] and dexetimide[103], labelled with radio-iodine, have demonstrated, in *in vitro* and *in vivo* animal experiments, high affinities and selectivities. Due to the slow cerebral uptake of iodo-QNB (IQNB), SPECT images of the brain's specific binding of [123]I-IQNB have been generally obtained 15 h after the administration of the racemic tracer[32]. Yet, in selecting carefully the isomer used (IQNB has four diastereoisomers with different affinities and different kinetics) it should be possible to define appropriate imaging protocols[28]. Preliminary. results in patients with dementia (Alzheimer's and Pick's diseases) have shown a constant reduced uptake in focal areas (frontal and parietal cortices) but an increased uptake in non-atrophic cortical areas[100]. Alzheimer's disease involves selective loss of $M_2$, but not $M_1$, muscarinic receptor subtypes. [123]I-IQNB binds equally to $M_1$ and $M_2$ receptors, however by taking advantage of the different pharmacokinetic properties of the (R-R) isomer for the $M_1$ and the $M_2$ subtypes, it should be possible to estimate losses in the $M_2$ receptor[107].

A halogenated dexetimide analogue, [123]I-iododexetimide, has demonstrate in mice appropriate pharmacological properties (*in vivo* receptor saturability and stereospecificity) to be potentially useful for imaging muscarinic cholinergic receptors in the living human brain[62,97,103]. Using the radiolabelled biologically inactive stereoisomer, iodolevetimide, it has been possible to quantitate the nonspecific part of [123]I-iododexetimide binding. Substraction of [123]I-iodolevetimide from [123]I-iododexetimide images on a pixel-to-pixel basis therefore reflects [123]I-iododexetimide specific binding to muscarinic receptors. This use of stereoisomerism to directly assess non-specific binding of [123]I-dexetimide has allowed successful imaging of muscarinic receptors in humans[73].

Despite relatively high non-specific binding, [123]I-dexetimide might also be useful in SPECT imaging of myocardial muscarinic receptors[62].

## GABAergic system

### *Benzodiazepine binding sites*

GABA is considered to be the most important inhibitory neurotransmitter in the mammalian central nervous system. The benzodiazepine receptor is part of the $GABA_A$ macromolecular complex that is coupled to a chloride channel. Benzodiazepines do not have direct actions on their own but act solely by enhancing the ability of GABA to increase the permeability of the ionophore.

In the mammalian brain, two different benzodiazepine binding sites, the central (neurons) and the peripheral types (glial cells) have been characterized[10,83]. However, only the central type has been extensively investigated due to its ubiquitous distribution and clinical importance.

## Peripheral type

Preliminary *in vivo* autoradiographic studies of brain with [125]I-labelled analogue of PK 11195, performed in experimental glioma-bearing rats, have suggested that this iodinated ligand could be a useful tracer for the visualization of peripheral benzodiazepine binding sites[29]. Its potential application to investigate brain tumours (gliomas) has not yet been established.

## Central type

For SPECT imaging, several iodinated benzodiazepine ligands have been prepared: iodoflunitrazepam[106], quinolin derivatives[58], iomazenil or Ro-16-0154. Iomazenil, the iodo analogue of the antagonist flumazenil[3] in which the 8-fluorine atom has been substituted by a 7-iodine atom has been shown to bind to brain tissue homogenates in a reversible, saturable, and highly specific way. Biodistribution of [123]I-iomazenil in non-human[35,93] and human[31] primate brain was found to parallel the known distribution of benzodiazepine receptors. Dynamic SPECT acquisition performed in humans has demonstrated that this ligand possesses the favourable physical characteristics for subsequent compartmental analysis: saturability (90 per cent of the brain radioactivity can be displaced by intravenous administration of benzodiazepine specific ligands), high initial brain uptake and slow wash-out rate[104]. In the baboon [123]I-iomazenil has been used as a SPECT probe for *in vivo* radioreceptor assays. As the uptake of this radioligand was relatively stable for several hours, a determination of the *in vivo* potency ($IC_{50}$) of any cold competitive drug acting at the benzodiazepine receptor could be performed from one scanning session in which stepwise increasing doses of the displacer were administered[36]. Altered distribution of [123]I-iomazenil was demonstrated in partial epilepsy[85]. In patients with medically intractable complex partial seizures, [123]I-iomazenil and SPECT was considered for the identification of the epileptic focus during the interictal phase. The results were correct in 85 per cent of the cases, a figure which is far higher than those obtained with SPECT blood flow measurements and comparable with those obtained with [18]F-FDG and PET. A theoretical advantage of [123]I-iomazenil is that it appears to reflect specifically changes in the functioning of membranes of neurons, whereas [18]F-FDG is related to glucose metabolism of both neurons and glial cells[98].

## Other systems

### Opioid receptors

[123]I-iodomorphine was applied via intracerebroventricular administration in patients treated by morphinotherapy. Gamma-scintigraphy images showed only a slight diffusion of the iodinated molecule beyond the ventricular system[94].

's' binding sites are supposed to play a role in mediating the antipsychotic effects of typical and atypical neuroleptic drugs. Preliminary *in vitro* and *in vivo* pharmacological studies have shown that new classes of iodinated compounds such as the derivatives of pyrrolidinyl ethylamine and of ethylpiperazine[20] and of di-*o*-tolylguanidine[46] are potential SPECT ligands for the s-receptors.

### NMDA receptor complex

MK-801 is a potent non-competitive NMDA receptor antagonist possessing anticonvulsant and neuroprotective actions. [123]I-iodo-MK-801 specifically labels the NMDA receptor complex *in vitro*, in rat brain membranes[77]. As this tracer binds preferentially to the activated state of the receptor, it could be a sensitive probe for SPECT imaging.

## Commentary

Progress in nuclear medicine relies principally on two factors: development of new, highly specific tracers and improvements in the quality of imaging devices. The somewhat inexpensive SPECT imaging technique that is mostly used for CBF measurement is also a promising technique for the clinical investigation of brain neurotransmission. Several $^{123}$I-labelled receptor ligands are currently under development. If these ligands meet expectations, we can hope that the increasing progress in single-photon quantitation available in tomographic instrumentation will soon make the clinical mapping and measurement of brain specific binding sites possible. In these conditions, SPECT will become a valuable diagnostic tool in the expanding field of brain imaging in neurology and psychiatry. Thus, at least for the dopaminergic and the benzodiazepine systems, some clinical evidence already supports the contention that *in vivo* receptor binding clinical studies provide a valuable addition to the nuclear medicine armamentorium.

# References

1.  Adam, M.J., Zea Ponce, Y., Berry, J.M. & Hoy, J.K. (1990): Synthesis and preliminary evaluation of L-$^{123}$I-iododopa as a potential SPECT brain imaging agent. *J. Label. Compound. Radiopharmacol.* **28**, 155–166.

2.  Basmadjian, G.P., Jain, S., Mills, S.L., Leonard, J.C. & Kanvinde, M.H. (1991): Carrier free radioiodinated cocaine: synthesis and animal biodistribution. *J. Nucl. Med.* **5**, 965 (abstr.)

3.  Beer, H.F., Blauenstein, P., Hasler, P.H., Delaloye, B., Riccabona, G., Bangerl, I., Hunkeler, W., Bonetti, E.P. Richards, J.G. & Bonetti, E.P. (1990): *In vitro* and *in vivo* evaluation of $^{123}$I-Ro-16-0154: a new imaging agent for SPECT investigations of benzodiazepine receptors. *J. Nucl. Med.* **31**, 1007–1014.

4.  Beer, H.F., Lin, S., Novak-Hoffer, I., Blauenstein, P. & Schubiger, P.A. (1992): Large scale preparation strategy for labelling of $^{123}$I-SCH 23982, a dopamine D$_1$ receptor binding agent. *Appl. Radiat. Isot.* **46**, 781–787.

5.  Billings, J., Kung, M.-P, Chumpradit, S., Pan, S. & Kung, H.F. (1989): $^{125}$I(+/-)FISCH: A new CNS D$_1$ dopamine receptor imaging ligand. *Life Sci.* **45**, 711–718.

6.  Billings, J.J., Kung, M.-P, Chumpradit, S., Mozley, D., Alavi, A. & Kung, H.F. (1992): Characterization of radioiodinated TISCH: A high affinity and selective ligand for mapping CNS D1 dopamine receptor. *J. Neurochem.* **58**, 227–236.

7.  Bloom, F.E. (1988): Neurotransmitters: past, present,and future directions. *FASEB J.* **2**, 32–41.

8.  Boja, J.W., Patel, A., Carroll, F.Y., Rahman, M.A., Philip, A., Lewin, A.H., Kopajtic, T.A. & Kuhar, M.J. (1991): [$^{125}$I]RTI-55: a potent ligand for dopamine transporters. *J. Pharmacol.* **194**, 133–134.

9.  Bossuyt, A., Mertens, J., Piron-Bossuyt, C. & Gijsemans, M. (1989): Mapping of serotonin S2 receptor sites by means of I-ketanserin. In: *Radio iodinated molecules for in vivo receptor mapping with SPECT*, eds. J. Mertens & C. Bossuyt-Piron. Brussels: Vrije University Press.

10. Braestrup, C. & Squires, R.F. (1977): Specific benzodiazepine receptors in rat brain characterized by high affinity [$^3$H]diazepam binding. *Proc. Natl. Acad. Sci. USA* **74**, 3805–3809.

11. Breese, G.R. & Creese, I. eds. (1986): *Neurobiology of central D1 dopamine receptors.* New York: Plenum Press.

12. Brücke, T., Podreka, I., Angelberger, P., Wenger, S., Topitz, A. Küfferle, B., Müller, Ch. & Deeke, L. (1991): Dopamine D2 receptor imaging with SPECT: Studies in different neuropsychiatric disorders. *J. Cereb. Blood Flow Metab.* **11**, 220–228.

13. Cantineau, R., Damhaut, P., Plenevaux, A., Lemaire, C. & Guillaume, M. (1991): Synthesis and preliminary animal studies of $^{131}$I-iodotropapride: a cerebral dopamine D2 receptor ligand. *J. Label. Comp. RadiopharmACOL.* **30**, 360–361.

14. Chabriat, H., Levasseur, M., Vidaiher, M., Loc'h, C. Mazière, B., Bourguignon, M., Bonnet, A.M., Zilbovicius, M., Raynaud, C., Agid, Y., Syrota, A. & Samson, Y. (1992): *In vivo* SPECT imaging of D2 receptor with $^{123}$I-iodolisuride. Results in supranuclear palsy. *J. Nucl. Med.* **23**, 1481–1485.

15. Chalon, S., Guimbal, C., Guilloteau, D., Mayo, W., Huguet, F., Schmitt, M.-H., Desplanches, G., Gaulieu, J.-L. & Besnard, J.-C. (1990): Iodobenzamide for *in vivo* exploration of central dopamine receptors: evaluation in animal models of supersensitivity. *Life Sci.* **47**, 729–734.

16.    Chiron, C., Bulteau, C., Loc'h, C., Raynaud, C., Mazière, B., de la Caffinière, H., Launay, J.K.M., Garreau, B., Leroy-Willig, A. & Syrota, A. (1993): Dopaminergic D2 receptor SPECT imaging in Rett syndrome: increase of specific binding in striatum. *J. Nucl. Med.* (In press)

17.    Chiueh, C.C., Bruecke, T., Singhaniyom, W., McLellan, C., Tsai, T., Cohen, R.M. & Kung, H.F. (1988): Preclinical trial of a SPECT imaging ligand for denervation-induced supersensitive D2 dopamine receptors: [123]I-labelled benzamide (IBZM). *J. Nucl. Med.* **29**, 759.

18.    Chumpradit, S., Kung, H.F., Billings, J., Kung, M.-P. & Pan, S. (1989:. (+/-)-7-Chloro-8-hydroxy-1-(4' [125]I-iodophenyl)-3-methyl-2,3,4,5-tetrahydro-1H-3-benzazepine: a potential CNS D1 dopamine receptor imaging agent. *J. Med. Chem.* **32**, 1431–1435.

19.    Costa, D.C., Verhoeff, N.P.L.G., Cullum, I.D., Ell, P.J., Syed, G.M.S., Barret, J., Palazidou, E., Toone, B., Van Royen, E. & Bobeldijk, M. (1990): *In vivo* characterisation of 3-iodo-6-methoxybenzamide [123]I in humans. *Eur. J. Nucl. Med.* **16**, 813–816.

20.    Decosta, B.L., Radesca, C., Dominguez, L., Dipaolo, L. & Bowen, W.D. (1992): Synthesis of fluoro-substituted and iodo-substituted high affinity sigma-receptor ligands – identification of potential PET and SPECT sigma-receptor imaging agents. *J. Med. Chem.* **35**, 2221–2230.

21.    Eckelman, W.C., Eng, R., Rzeszotarski, W.J., Gibson, R.E., Francis, B. & Reba, R.C. (1985): Use of 3-quinuclidinyl 4-iodobenzylate as a receptor binding radiotracer. *J. Nucl. Med.* **26**, 637–642.

22.    Efange, S.M.N., Dutta, A.K., Michelson, R.H., Kung, H.F., Thomas, J.R., Billings, J. & Boudreau, R.J. (1992): Radioiodinated 2-hydroxy-3-(4-iodophenyl)-1-(4-phenylpiperidinyl) propane: potential radiotracer for mapping cholinergic innervation *in vivo*. *Nucl. Med. Biol.* **19**, 337–348.

23.    Engel, G., Muller-Schweinitzer, E. & Palacios, J.M. (1984): 2-[125]I-iodo-LSD, a new ligand for the characterisation and localisation of 5-HT2 receptors. *Naunyn Schmiedeberg's Arch. Pharmacol.* **325**, 328–336.

24.    Farde, L. (1992): Selective D1 and D2 dopamine receptor blockade both induces akathisia in humans – a PET study with [11]C-SCH23390 and [11]C-raclopride. *Psychopharmacol.* **107**, 23–29.

25.    Foulon, C., Garreau, L., Chalon, S., Desplanches, G., Frangin, Y., Besnard, J.-C. & Guilloteau, D. (1992): Synthesis and *in vitro* binding properties of halogenated analogues of GBR as new dopamine uptake carrier ligands. *Nucl. Med. Biol.* **19**, 597–600.

26.    Frost, J.J., Smith, A.C., Kuhar, M.J., Dannals, R.F. & Wagner, H.N. (1987): *In vivo* binding of [3]H-N-methylspiperone to dopamine and serotonin receptors. *Life Sci.* **40**, 987–995.

27.    Geaney, D.P., Ellis, P.M., Soper, N., Shepstone, B.J. & Cowen, P.J. (1992): Single photon emission tomography assessment of cerebral dopamine D2 receptor blockade in schizophrenia. *Biol. Psychiatry* **32**, 293–295.

28.    Gibson, R.E., Schneidau, T.A., Cohen, V.I., Sood, V., Ruch, J., Melograna, J., Eckelman, W.C. & Reba, R.C. (1989): *In vitro* and *in vivo* characteristics of [125]Iodine-3-(R)-quinuclidinyl (S)-4-iodobenzylate. *J. Nucl. Med.* **30**, 1079–1087.

29.    Gildersleeve, D.L., Lin, T.-Y., Wieland, D.M., Ciliax, B.J., Olson, J.M.M. & Young, A.B. (1989): Synthesis of a high specific activity [125]I-labelled analogue of PK11195, potential agent for SPECT imaging of the peripheral benzodiazepine binding site. *Nucl. Med. Biol.* **16**, 423–429.

30.    Hall, H., Höggberg, T., Halldin, C., Köhler, C., Dtröm, P., Ross, S.B., Larsson, S.A. & Farde, L. (1991): NCQ 298, a new selective iodinated salicylamide ligand for the labelling of dopamine D2 receptors. *Psychopharmacology* **103**, 6–18.

31.    Holl, K., Deisenhammer, E., Dauth, J., Carmann, H. & Schubiger, P.A. (1989): Imaging benzodiazepine receptors in the human brain by single photon emission tomography (SPECT). *Nucl. Med. Biol.* **16**, 759–763.

32.    Holman, B.L., Gibson, R.E., Hill, T.C., Eckelman W.C., Albert, M. & Reba, R.C. (1985): Muscarinic acetylcholine receptors in Alzheimer's disease. *In vivo* imaging with [123]I-labeled 3-quinuclidinyl-4-iodobenzylate and emission tomography. *J.A.M.A.* **254**, 3063–3066.

33.    Humphreys, C.J., Cassel, D. & Rudnick, G. (1989): 2-Iodoimiprimine, a novel ligand for the serotonin transporter. *Mol. Pharmacol.* **36**, 620–626.

34.    Innis, R., Baldwin, R., Sybirska, E., Zea, Y., Laruelle, M., Al-Tikriti, M., Cjarney, D. Zoghbi, S., Smith, E., Wisnievski, G., Hoffer, P., Wang, S., Millius, R. & Neumeyer, J. (1991): Single photon emission computed tomography imaging of monoamine reuptake sites in primate brain with [123]I-CIT. *Eur. J. Pharmacol.* **200**, 369–370.

35.    Innis, R., Zoghbi, S., Johnson, E., Woods, S., Al-Tikriti, M., Baldwin, R., Seibyl, J., Malison, R., Zubal, G., Charney, D., Heninger, G. & Hoffer, P. (1991): SPECT imaging of the benzodiazepine receptor in non-human primate brain with [123]I-Ro 16-0154. *Eur. J. Pharmacol.* **193**, 249–252.

36.    Innis, R., Al-Tikriti, M., Zoghbi, S.S., Baldwin, R., Sybirska, E.H., Laruelle, M.A., Malison, R.T., Seibyl, J.P., Zimmerman, R.C., Johnson, E.W., Smith, E.O., Charney, D.S., Heninger, G.R., Woods, S.W. & Hoffer, P.B. (1991): SPECT imaging of the benzodiazepine receptor: feasibility of the *in vivo* potency measurements from stepwise displacement curves. *J. Nucl. Med.* **32**, 1754–1761.

37.    Innis, R.B., Malison, R.T., Al-Tikriti, M., Hoffer, P., Sybirska, E.H., Seybil, J.P., Zoghbi, S.S., Baldwin, R.M., Laruelle, M., Smith, E.O., Charney, D.S., Heninger, G., Elsworth, J.D. & Roth, R.H. (1992): Amphetamine-stimulated dopamine release competes *in vivo* for $^{123}$I-IBZM binding to the D2 receptor in nonhuman primates. *Synapse* **10**, 177–184.

38.    Janowski, A., De Paulis, T., Clanton, J.A., Smith, H.E., Ebert, M.H. & Kessler, R.M. (1988): $^{125}$I-iodopride: a specific high affinity radioligand for labelling striatal dopamine D2 receptors. *Eur. J. Pharmacol.* **150**, 203–205.

39.    Jones, T. (1980): Positron emission tomography and measurements of regional tissue function in man. *Br. Med. Bull.* **36**, 231–236.

40.    Joyce, J.N., Janowsky, A. & Neve, K.A. (1991): Characterization and distribution of $^{125}$I-epidepride binding to dopamine D2 receptors in basal ganglia and cortex of human brain. *J. Pharmacol. Exp. Ther.* **257**, 1253–1263.

41.    Jung, Y.-W., Van Dort, M.E., Gildersleeve, D.L. & Wieland, D.M. (1990): A radiotracer for mapping cholinergic neurons of the brain. *J. Med. Chem.* **33**, 2065–2068.

42.    Kebabian, J.W. & Calne, D.B. (1979): Multiple receptors for dopamine. *Nature* **277**, 953–961.

43.    Kessler, R.M., Ansari, S., Schmidt, D.E., de Paulis, T., Clanton, J.A., Innis, R., Al-Tikriti, M., Manning, R.G. & Gillespie, D. (1991): High affinity dopamine D2 receptor radioligands. [$^{125}$I]Epidepride, a potent and specific radioligand for the characterization of striatal and extrastriatal dopamine D2 receptors. *Life Sci.* **49**, 617–628.

44.    Kessler, R.M., Mason, S.M., Votaw, J.R., De Paulis, T., Clanton, J.A., Sib Ansari, M. Schmidt, D.E., Manning, R.G. & Bell, R.L. (1992): Visualization of extrastriatal dopamine D2 receptors in the human brain. *Eur. J. Pharmacol.* **223**, 105–107.

45.    Kilbourn, M.R., Jung, Y.-W., Haka, M.S., Gildersleeve, D.L., Kuhl, D.E. & Wieland, D.M. (1990): Mouse brain distribution of carbon-11 labelled vesamicol derivative: presynaptic marker of cholinergic neurons. *Life Sci.* **47**, 1955–1963.

46.    Kimes, A.S., Wilson, A.A., Scheffel, U., Campbell, B.G. & London, E.D. (1992): Radiosynthesis, cerebral distribution, and binding of $^{125}$I-1-(*p*-iodophenyl)-3-(1-adamantyl)guanidine, a ligand for s binding sites. *J. Med. Chem.* **35**, 4683–4689.

47.    Kung, H.F., Guo, Y.-Z. & Billings, J.B. (1986): New serotonin receptor-site specific brain imaging agent, radioactive iodinated 8-OH-PAT. *J. Nucl. Med.* **27**, 972.

48.    Kung, H.F., Alavi, A., Billings, J.B., Kung, M.-P., Pan, S. & Reilly, J. (1988): $^{123}$I-IBZP: a potential CNS D1 dopamine receptor imaging agent, *in vivo* biodistribution in a monkey. *J. Nucl. Med.* **29, 758.**

49.    Kung, H.F., Pan, S., Kung, M.P. Billings, J., Kasliwal, R., Reilly, J. & Alavi, A. (1989): *In vitro* and *in vivo* evaluation of $^{123}$I-IBZM: A potential CNS D-2 dopamine receptor imaging agent. *J Nucl. Med.* **30,** 88–92.

50.    Kung, M.-P., Kung, H.F., Billings, J., Yang, Y., Murphy, R.A. & Alavi, A.(1990): The characterization of IBF as a new selective dopamine D2 receptor imaging agent. *J. Nucl. Med.* **31**, 648–654.

51.    Kung, M.-P., Chumpradit, S., Billings, J. & Kung, H. (1992): 4-Iodotomoxetine: a novel ligand for serotonin uptake sites. *Life Sci.* **51**, 95–106.

52.    Langley, J.N. (1905): On the reaction of cells and of nerve-endings to certain poisons, chiefly as regards the reaction of striatal muscle to nicotine and to curare. *J. Physiol.* **33**, 374.

53.    Lever, J.R., Scheffel, U.A., Stathis, M., Musachio, J.L. & Wagner Jr, H.N. (1990): *In vitro* and *in vivo* binding of (E)-and (Z)-(iodoallyl): spiperone to dopamine D2 and serotonin 5-HT2 neororeceptors. *Life Sci.* **46**, 1967–1976.

54.    Lever, J.R., Scheffel, U.A., Musachio, J.L., Stathis, M. & Wagner Jr, H.N. (1991). Radioiodinated D-(+)-N1-ethyl-2-iodolysergic acid diethylamide: a ligand for *in vitro* and *in vivo* studies of serotonin receptors. *Life Sci.* **48**, 73–78.

55.    Loc'h, C., Mazière, B., Raynaud, C., Bourguignon, M., Hantraye, P., Stulzaft, O., Syrota, A & Mazière, M. (1989): SPECT imaging of dopaminergic D2 receptors with $^{123}$I-iodolisuride (123-I-ILIS). *Eur. J. Nucl. Med.* **15**, 403.

56.    Loc'h, C., Guillaume, M., Mazière, B., Brutesco, C., Bourguignon, M., Bottlaender, M., Syrota, A. & Mazière, M. (1993): Radiohalogenic derivatives of tropapride for PET and SPECT investigations of the dopamine D2 receptors. *J. Nucl. Med.* in press.

57.     Macwhorter, S.E. & Baldwin, R.M. (1991): Synthesis and biodistribution of N-(2-aminoethyl)-5-iodo-2-pyridinecarboxamide (Ro 43-0463), a monoamine oxidase B inhibitor. *Nucl. Med. Biol.* **18**, 563–564.

58.     Maeda, M., Komori, H., Dohmoto, H. & Kojima M. (1985): Synthesis of radioiodinated analogs of 2-phenyl pyrazolo [4,3]-quinolin-3 (5H)-one by a modified triazene method. *J. Label. Compound Radiopharmacol.* **22**, 487–501.

59.     Martres, M.-P., Salès, N., Bouthenet, M.-L. & Schwartz J.-C. (1985): Localization and pharmacological characterization of D2 dopamine receptors in rat cerebral neocortex and cerebellum using [125]I-iodosulpride. *Eur. J. Pharmacol.* **118**, 211–219.

60.     Mathis, C.A., Gerdes, J.M., Enas, J.D., Havlik, S. & Peroutka, S.J. (1991): [125]I-iodoparoxetine: synthesis and preliminary evaluation of a presynaptic serotonin ligand. *J. Nucl. Med.* **32**, 965.

61.     Mathis, C.A., Biegon, A., Taylor, S.E., Enas, J.D. & Hanrahan, S.M. (1992): [125]I-5-Iodo-6-nitro-2-piperazinylquinoline: a potent and selective ligand for the serotonin uptake complex. *Eur. J. Pharmacol,* **210**, 103–104.

62.     Matsumura, K., Uno, Y., Scheffel, U., Wilson, A.A., Dannals, R.F. & Wagner H.N. (1991): *In vitro* and *in vivo* characterization of 4-[123]I-iododexetimide binding to muscarinic cholinergic receptors in rat heart. *J. Nucl. Med.* **32**, 76–80.

63.     Mazière, B., Loc'h, C., Raynaud, C., Hantraye, P., Stulzaft, O., Syrota, A. & Mazière, M. (1989): [123]I-iodolisuride, a new SPECT imaging ligand for brain dopamine D2 receptors. *J. Nucl. Med.* **30**, 731.

64.     Mazière, B. & Mazière, M. (1990): Where have we got with neuroreceptor mapping? *Eur. J. Nucl. Med.* **16,** 817–835.

65.     Mckenna, D.J., Nazarali, A.J., Hoffman, A.J., Nichols, D.R., Mathis, C.A. & Saavedra, J.M. (1989): Common receptors for hallucinogens in rat brain: a comparative autoradiographic study using [125]I-LSD and [125]I-DOI, a new psychomimetic radioligand. *Brain Res.* **476**, 45–56

66.     McQuade, R.D., Chipkin, R., Amlaiky, N., Caron, M., Ioro, L. & Barnett, A. (1988): Characterization of the radioiodinated analogue of SCH 23390: *in vitro* and *in vivo* D1 dopamine receptor binding studies. *Life Sci.* **43**, 1151–1216.

67.     Mertens, J., Terriere, D., Bossuyt, A. & Bossuyt-Piron C. (1988): 4-[123]I-spiperone of high purity and high specific activity, a suitable tracer for imaging dopamine receptors sites in baboon brains with SPECT. In: *Seventh International Symposium on Radiopharmaceutical Chemistry*, ed. W. Vaalburg, pp. 135–136. University of Groningen.

68.     Mertens, J., Bossuyt-Piron, C., De Geeter, F., Christiaens, L., Cantineau, R., Guillaume, M. & Leyssen, J. (1989): Evaluation of pure 2'-[123]I-spiperone as a promising tracer for *in vivo* receptor studies with SPECT. *J. Nucl. Med.* **30**, 926.

69.     Mertens, J., Bossuyt-Piron, C., Guns, M., Bossuyt, A. & Leysen, J. (1989): High selective serotonin S2 receptor mapping with SPECT in baboon brain. *J. Nucl. Med.* **30**, 741.

70.     Mertens, J., Gysemans, M., Bossuyt-Piron, C. & Thomas, M. (1990): High yield preparation of pure 2-radioiodo-ketanserin of high specific activity, a serotonin S2 receptor tracer for SPECT. *J. Label. Compound Radiopharmacol.* **28**, 731–738.

71.     Metwally, S.A.M., Gatley, S.J., Wolf, A.P. & Yu, D.W. (1992): Synthesis and binding to striatal membranes of no carrier added [123]I-labelled-iodococaine. *J. Label. Compound Radiopharmacol.* **31**, 219–225.

72.     Mozley, P.D., Zhu, X.W., Kung, H.F., Selikson, M.H., Hickey, J., Galloway, S., Pfieffer, N. & Alavi, A. (1993): The dosimetry of iodine-123-labelled TISCH. A SPECT imaging agent for the D1 dopamine receptor. *J. Nucl. Med.* **34**, 208–213.

73.     Müller-Gartner, H.-W., Wilson, A.A., Dannals, R.F., Wagner, H.N. & Frost, J.J. (1992): Imaging muscarinic receptors in human brain *in vivo* with SPECT, [123]I-4-iododexetimide and [123]I-4-iodolevetimide. *J. Cereb. Blood Flow Metab.* **12**, 562–570.

74.     Neumeyer, J.L., Wang, S., Milius, R.A., Baldwin, R.M., Zea-Ponce, Y., Hoffer, P.B., Sybirska, E., Al-Tikriti, M., Charney, D.S., Malison, R.T., Laruelle, M., & Innis, R.B. (1991): [[123]I]-2-carbomethoxy-3-(4-iodophenyl)-tropane: high affinity SPECT radiotracer of monoamine reuptake sites in the brain. *J. Med. Chem.* **34**, 3144–3146.

75.     Ohmono, Y., Hirata, M., Murakami, K., Magata, Y., Tanaka, C. & Yokohama, A. (1991): Synthesis of fluorine and iodine analogues of clorgyline and selective inhibition of monoamine oxidase-A. *Chem. Pharm. Bull.* **39**, 1038–1040.

76.    Pilowski, L.S., Costa, D.C., Ell, P.J., Murray, R.M., Verhoeff, N.P. & Kerwin, R.W. (1992): Clozapine, single photon emission tomography and the D2 dopamine receptor blockade hypothesis. *Lancet* **340**, 199–202.

77.    Ransom, R.W., Eng, W., Burns, H.D., Gibson, R.E. & Solomon, H.F. (1990): (+)-3-[123]I-iodo-MK-801: synthesis and characterization of binding to the *N*-methyl-D-aspartate receptor complex. *Life Sci.* **46**, 1103–1110.

78.    Saji, H., Nakatsuka, I., Shiba, K., Tokui, T., Horiuchi, K., Yoshitake, A., Torizuka, K. & Yokoyama, A. (1987): Radioiodinated 2'-iodospiperone: a new radioligand for *in vivo* dopamine receptor study. *Life Sci.* **41**, 1999–2006.

79.    Saji, H., Iida, Y., Magata, Y., Yonekura, Y., Iwasaki, Y., Sasayama, S., Kopnishi, J., Nakaatsuka, I., Shiba, K., Yoshitake, A. & Yokoyama, A. (1992): Preparation of [123]I-labeled 2'-iodospiperone and imaging of D2 dopamine receptors in the human brain using SPECT. *Nucl. Med. Biol.* **19**, 523–529.

80.    Saji, H., Tokui, T., Nakatsuka, I., Saiga, A., Magata, Y., Shiba, K., Yoshitake, A. & Yokoyama, A. (1992): Evaluation of *N*-alkyl derivatives of radioiodinated spiperone as radioligands for *in vivo* dopamine D2 receptors studies: effects of lipophilicity and receptor affinity on the *in vivo* biodistribution. *Chem. Pharm. Bull.* **40**, 165–169.

81.    Sanchez-Roa, P.M., Grigoriadis, D.E., Wilson, A.A., Sharkey, J., Dannals, R.F., Villemagne, V.L., Wong, D.F., Wagner, H.N. & Kuhar, M. (1989): [125]I-spectramide: a novel benzamide displaying potent and selective effects at the D2 dopamine receptor. *Life Sci.* **45**, 1821–1829.

82.    Scheffel, U., Dannals, R.F., Cline, E.J., Ricaurte, G.A., Caroll, F.I., Abraham, P., Lewin, A.H. & Kuhar, M.J. (1992): [123/125]I-RTI-55, an *in vivo* label for the serotonin transporter. *Synapse* **11**, 134–139.

83.    Schoemaker, H., Boles, R.G., Horst, W.D. & Yamamura, H.I. (1983): Specific high-affinity binding sites for [[3]H]Ro 5-4864 in rat brain and kidney. *J. Pharmacol. Exp. Ther.* **225**, 61–69.

84.    Schotte, A. & Leysen J.E. (1989): Identification of 5-HT2 receptors, α-adrenoreceptors and amine release sites in rat brain by autoradiography with [125]I-7-amino-8-iodo-ketanserin. *Eur. J. Pharmacol. Mol. Sect.* **172**, 99–106.

85.    Schubiger, P.A., Hasler, P.H., Beer-Wohlfahrt, H., Bekier, A., Oettli, R., Cordes, M., Ferstl, F., Deisenhammer, E., De Roo, M., Moser, E., Nitzsche, E., Podreka, I., Riccabona, G., Bangerl, I., Schober, O., Bartenstein, P., Van Rijk, P., Van Isselt, J.W., Van Royen, E.A., Verhoeff, N.P. Haldemann, R. & Von Svhulthess, G.K. (1991): Evaluation of a multicentre study with iomazenil – a benzodiazepine receptor ligand. *Nucl. Med. Comm.* **12**, 569–582.

86.    Schwarz, J., Tatsch, K., Vogl, T., Kirsch, C.-M., Trenkwalder, C., Arnold, G., Gasser, T. & Oertel, W.H. (1992): Marked reduction of striatal dopamine-D2 receptors as detected by [123]I-IBZM-SPECT in a Wilson's disease patient with generalized dystonia. *Mov. Disorders* **7**, 58–61.

87.    Schwarz, J., Tatsch, K., Vogl, T., Arnold, G., Gasser, T., Trenkwalder, C., Kirsch, C.-M. & Oertel, W.H. (1992): [123]I-iodobenzamide-SPECT predicts dopaminergic responsiveness in patients with *de novo* parkinsonism. *Neurology* **42**, 556–561.

88.    Seibyl, J.P., Woods, S.W., Zoghbi, S.S., Baldwin, R.M., Dey, H.M., Goddard, A.W., Zea-Ponce, Y., Zubla, G., Germine, M., Smith, E.O., Heninger, G.R., Charney, D.S., Kung, H.F., Alavi, A., Hoffer, P.B. & Innis R.B. (1992): Dynamic SPECT imaging of dopamine D2 receptors in human subjects with iodine-123-IBZM. *J. Nucl. Med.* **33**, 1964–1971.

89.    Shaya, E.K., Scheffel, U., Dannals, R.F., Ricaurta, G.A., Caroll, F.Y., Wagner, H.N., Kuhar, M..J. & Wong, D.F. (1992): *In vivo* imaging of dopamine reuptake sites in the primate brain using single photon emission tomography (SPECT) and iodine-123-labelled RTI55. *Synapse,* **10**, 169–172.

90.    Sidhu, A., Van Oene, J.C., Dandridge, P., Kaiser, C. & Kebebian, J.W. (1986): [125]I-SCH 23982: the ligand of choice for identifying the D1 dopamine receptor. *Eur. J. Pharmacol.* **128**, 213–220.

91.    Stoof, J.C. & Kebabian, J.W. (1981): Opposing roles for D1 and D2 dopamine receptors in efflux of cyclic AMP from rat neostriatum. *Nature* **294**, 366–368.

92.    Stoof, J.C. & Kebabian J.W. (1984): Two dopamine receptors. Biochemistry, physiology and pharmacology. *Life Sci.* **35**, 2281–2296.

93.    Sybirska, E., Al-Tikriti, M., Zoghbi, S.S., Baldwin, R.M., Johnson, E.W. & Innis, R.B. (1992): SPECT imaging of the benzodiazepine receptor – autoradiographic comparison of receptor density and radioligand distribution. *Synapse* **12**, 119–128.

94.     Tafani, J.A.M., Lazorthes, Y., Danet, B., Verdie, J.C., Esquerre, J.P. Simon, J. & Guiraud, R.(1989:. Human brain and spinal cord scan after intracerebroventricular administration of iodine-123 morphine. *Nucl. Med. Biol.* **16**, 505–509.

95.     Tatsch, K., Schwarz, J., Oertel, W.H. & Kirsch C.-M. (1991): SPECT imaging of dopamine D2 receptors with [123]I-IBZM: initial experience in controls and patients with Parkinson's syndrome and Wilson's disease. *Nucl. Med. Comm.* **12**, 699–707.

96.     Thonoor, C.M., Couch, M.W., Greer, D.M., Thomas, K.D. & Williams, C.M. (1988): Biodistribution and radiation dosimetry of radioiodinated-SCH 23982, a potential dopamine D1 receptor imaging agent. *J. Nucl. Med.* **29**, 1668–1674.

97.     Uno, Y., Matsazmura, K., Scheffel, U., Wilson, A.A., Dannals, R.F. & Wagner, H.N. (1991): Effects of atropine treatment on *in vitro* and *in vivo* binding of 4-[123]I-dexetimide to central and myocardial muscarinic receptors. *Eur. J. Nucl. Med.* **18**, 447–452.

98.     Van Huffelen, A.C., Van Isselt, J.W., Van Veelen, C.W., Van Rijk, P.P., Van Bentum, A.M., Dive, D., Maquet, P., Franck, G,, Velis, D.N., Van Emde Boas, W. & Debets, R.M. (1990): Identification of the side of the epileptic focus with [123]I-iomazenil SPECT. *Acta Neurochir. Suppl.* **50**, 95–99.

99.     Van der Krogt, J.A., Pauwels, E.K., Van Doremalen, P.A., Wijnhoven, G., Reiffers, S., Van Valkenburg, C.F. & Buruma, O.J. (1992): 4-[123]I-iodospiperone as a ligand for dopamine DA receptors: *in vitro* and *in vivo* experiments in a rat model. *Nucl. Med. Biol.* **19**, 759–763.

100.    Weinberger, D.R., Gibson, R.E., Coppola, R., Jones, D.W., Braun, A.R., Mann, U., Berman, K.F., Sunderland, T., Chase, T.N. & Reba, R.C. (1989): Distribution of muscarinic receptors in patients with dementia: a controlled study of [123]I-QNB and SPECT. *J. Cereb. Blood Flow Metab.* **9**, S537.

101.    Widen, L., Eriksson, L., Ingvar, M., Parsons, S.M., Rogers, G.A. & Stone-Elander, S. (1992): Positron emission tomographic studies of central cholinergic nerve terminals. *Neurosci. Lett.* **136**, 1–4.

102.    Wilson, A.A., Dannals, R.F., Hayden, D., Ravert, T. & Wagner, H.N. (1989): Preparation of [11]C- and [125]I-IMB: a dopamine D2 receptor antagonist. *Appl. Radiat. Isot.* **40**, 369–373.

103.    Wilson, A.A., Dannals, R.F., Ravert, H.T., Frost, J.J. & Wagner, Jr, H.N. (1989): Synthesis and biological evaluation of [125]I and [123]I-4-iododexetimide, a potent muscarinic cholinergic receptor antagonist. *J. Med. Chem.* **32**, 1057–1062.

104.    Woods, S.W., Seibyl, J.P., Goddard, A.W., Dey, H.M., Zoghbi, S.S., Germine, M., Baldwin, R.M., Smith, E.O., Charney, D.S., Heninger, G.R., Hoffer, P.B. & Innis, R.B. (1992): Dynamic SPECT imaging after injection of the benzodiazepine receptor ligand [123]I-iomazenil in healthy human subjects. *Psychiatry Res. Neuroimaging* **45**, 67–77.

105.    Yu, D.W, Gatley, S.J., Wolf, A.P., MacGregor, R.R., Dewey, S.L., Fowler, J.S. & Schyler, D.J. (1992): Synthesis of carbon-11-labelled iodinated cocaine derivatives and their distribution in baboon brain measured using positron emission tomography. *J. Med. Chem.* **35**, 2178–2183.

106.    Zecca, L. & Ferrario, P. (1988): Synthesis and biodistribution of an [123]I-labelled flunitrazepam derivative: a potential *in vivo* tracer for benzodiazepine receptors. *Appl. Radiat. Isot.* **39**, 353–356.

107.    Zeeberg, B.R., Kim, H.J. & Reba, R.C. (1992): Pharmacokinetic simulations of SPECT quantitation of the M2 muscarinic neuroreceptor subtype in diseases states using radioiodinated (R,R)-4 IQNB. *Life Sci.* **51**, 661–670.

# Section V
# CLINICAL APPLICATIONS

The ultimate goal in the development of new nuclear medicine methodologies is the potential for routine application in the early diagnosis and follow-up of diseases or monitorization of therapeutic measures.

At present, several modalities of neuroimaging complement each other in the investigation of patients with neuropsychiatric diseases. Whilst it is too early to establish adequate diagnostic neuroimaging organigrams, the following chapters demonstrate that there are already well identified clinical applications for the use of brain SPET. However, we still have a long way to go before the desired 'diagnostic neuroimaging trees' are achieved.

*New Trends in Nuclear Neurology and Psychiatry*, edited by D.C. Costa, G.F. Morgan and N. A. Lassen
© 1993 John Libbey & Company Ltd., pp. 103–117

# Chapter 7

## Clinical decision making and brain SPECT

I. Podreka, Th. Brücke, S. Asenbaum, S. Wenger, S. Aull, C. van der Meer and
Ch. Baumgartner

*Neurological University Clinic, Vienna, Austria*

SPECT in general is a useful tool for the clinical diagnosis and in some instances for therapeutic decisions in neurological diseases. Main indications for the visualization/calculation of cerebral blood flow (CBF) are stroke, partial seizures and processes leading to dementia. In stroke, repeated HMPAO-SPECT measurements can give prognostic information for the resolving of neurological symptoms. Combined investigations of CBF and cerebral blood volume (CBV) with radiolabelled red blood cells give insight into cerebral perfusion pressure in cases with stenoses of the carotid arteries. Another approach in assessing impaired cerebrovascular reactivity is the registration of CBF changes after acetazolamide administration or $CO_2$ inhalation. Both methods are used in candidates for surgical treatment of cerebrovascular disease. Surgical treatment of partial seizures resistant to anticonvulsive therapy has a clear-cut positive effect on seizure occurrence in properly selected patients. HMPAO-SPECT allows identification of the epileptogenic tissue volume in approximately 60–83 per cent and is performed routinely for noninvasive diagnosis of epilepsy and differential diagnosis of 'pseudo seizures'. Alzheimer's disease, multi-infarct dementia and Huntington's disease can be differentiated by HMPAO-SPECT. At present $D_2$ dopamine receptor studies are performed with iodobenzamide (IBZM). With this compound it is possible to differentiate between Parkinson's disease and multisystem atrophy. Early cases of Huntington's disease without morphological changes on MRI/CT can be diagnosed. Occupancy of $D_2$ dopamine receptors by various drugs is of great interest for the clinicians. It was shown that drugs like calcium channel blockers or specific neuroleptics block these receptors and therefore cause extrapyramidal symptoms. In such cases the decision of withdrawal from therapy, if possible, might be of benefit for the patient. Visualization of benzodiazepine receptors with iomazenil does not have at present any advantage in clinical decisions compared to CBF-SPECT.

## Introduction

The development of three dimensional imaging techniques has largely improved the possibilities of neurological diagnosis. While transmission computerized tomography (TCT) and magnetic resonance imaging (MRI) are used routinely for the detection of morphological lesions, imaging techniques with radiotracers such as positron emission tomography (PET) and single photon emission tomography (SPECT) should give insights into physiological processes and variables such as cerebral blood flow (CBF), brain metabolism (oxygen, glucose), protein synthesis in brain tissue, regional pH and others, or visualize various receptors in the brain in normal or pathological conditions. Considering the large numbers of these variables it is obvious that the clinical applicability of PET and SPECT is influenced very much by the research in the field of radiochemistry.

At present with SPECT it is only possible to visualize and/or measure cerebral blood flow (CBF) using a washout ($^{133}$Xe) or stable tracer technique (IMP, HMPAO, ECD). While the first allows quantification of hemispheric CBF and regional CBF (rCBF) in large tissue volumes, the latter offers a better delineation of rCBF also in subcortical brain structures, due to better counting statistics and spatial resolution. However, quantification of rCBF in absolute terms with these tracers is not yet possible, due to not fully elucidated tracer kinetics. Besides CBF, $D_2$ dopamine and benzodiazepine receptors can be visualized with SPECT after i.v. administration of iodobenzamide (IBZM) or iomazenil. In the following sections, we report on the present clinical usefulness of SPECT investigations in patients with neuropsychiatric disorders.

## Clinical application of SPECT

### Stroke

In several countries stroke is the third most frequent cause of death and therefore PET is used extensively for research in the field of cerebrovascular disease (CVD). It was shown by several groups that in acute stages of ischaemic stroke, CBF and glucose metabolism can be uncoupled. While CBF decreases, $CMRO_2$ and $CMR_{glu}$ can be preserved (stage termed as 'early mismatch'[33], or 'misery perfusion'[4]). At later stages CBF can be elevated beyond the metabolic demand ('luxury perfusion'[36]) with clearly depressed $CMRO_2$ or $CMR_{glu}$. Tissue underlying 'misery perfusion' may survive in the centre of ischaemia but most probably will become viable only at the border of the infarct ('penumbra')[5]. Usually in the core of an infarct CBF is reduced to values below 12 ml/100 g/min., while towards its periphery CBF increases to values above 18 ml/100 g/min. In the chronic stage of stroke (i.e. approximately more than 40 days after onset) CBF and metabolism are again coupled.

Now, which role can CBF measurement with SPECT have in CVD, although it does not directly provide any information on the metabolic situation? Based on the knowledge achieved by PET investigations, the CBF pattern obtained with SPECT in serial measurements can indirectly reveal the stage of stroke and the metabolic situation. Although absolute quantification of rCBF using brain perfusion tracers has not been fully achieved, some researchers have recently described[38,39] first pass protocols to calculate hemispheral CBF and from that the rCBF with SPECT.

Another method may be employed. By calculating the HMPAO-uptake/100 ml brain tissue it is possible to achieve information on CBF changes in the same individual. This can be accomplished quite easily since the injected amount of $^{99m}$Tc-HMPAO is known. By defining the brain boundaries manually or by automatic edge-finding the brain volume is obtained by summing up voxels of all reconstructed cross-sections within the established limits. The sum of the defined voxels multiplied by the single voxel volume gives the brain volume. However, attention must be paid in SPECT studies showing very 'hot' areas like a 'luxury perfusion' or highly increased rCBF during a partial seizure. Here, the separation limit of voxels which do and do not reflect brain tissue must be estimated carefully by the investigator, since an automatic cut-off limit would yield too small volumes. After SPECT-system calibration with an appropriate phantom, cts/voxel can be converted into µCi/voxel. Thus, the total HMPAO uptake in 'brain voxels' can be calculated and expressed as a percentage of the injected doses/100 ml brain tissue.

As was found in 20 subjects[43], in whom two SPECT studies separated by 7 days were performed, this procedure yields reproducible values for global HMPAO brain uptake (Fig. 1) ($r = 0.970$, $P < 0.001$), hemispheric HMPAO uptake (left hemisphere: $r = 0.962$, $P < 0.001$; right hemisphere: $r = 0.966$, $P < 0.001$) and HMPAO uptake in 34 ROIS (correlation coefficients between 0.902 and 0.976, all $P < 0.001$). However, the variability of values for global and hemispheric HMPAO

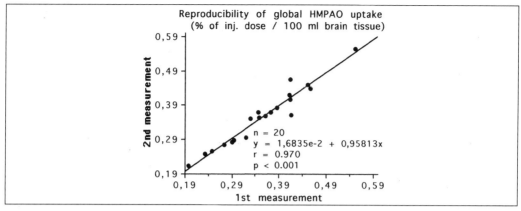

*Fig. 1. Correlation and regression obtained in repeated SPECT studies for global per cent-HMPAO brain uptake/100 ml in 20 subjects.*

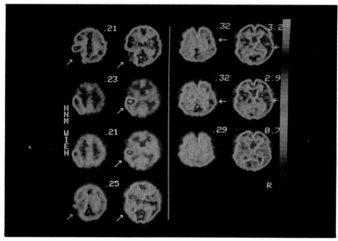

*Fig. 2. Four SPECT studies (1st two columns) obtained in Case A (47-year-old male patient). The first SPECT study was done approximately 20 h after onset of symptoms. A profound decrease of HMPAO uptake is seen in the left parietal and temporal region (arrows). This area is surrounded in central and frontal direction by a slightly increased tracer deposition. Seven (2nd row) and 14 days later (3rd row), a high HMPAO uptake is seen in the previously low perfused region. The last control SPECT study (29 days, 4th row) shows a decreased HMPAO deposition in the left parietal and temporal lobe as well as in the left central and latero-frontal region. Numbers indicate global per cent HMPAO uptake, which did not differ significantly through the studies. Columns 3 and 4 display three SPECT studies of Case B (female patient, 53 years of age). Images represent per cent HMPAO uptake; left number columns indicate global per cent HMPAO uptake/100 g, right columns per cent left/right asymmetry. In the first SPECT study (1 day after onset) a slight rightward asymmetry in hemispheric per cent HMPAO deposition was found (arrows), which was pronounced in the parietal and temporal region. As SPECT controls show (11 and 45 days after the insult), left/right per cent HMPAO uptake asymmetry decreased progressively to normal values. Global per cent HMPAO uptake did not change significantly.*

uptake can be in single cases 13–14 per cent, which is in the range of the variability obtained for $CMR_{glu}$ PET studies[40]. Regional HMPAO uptake values showed a higher variability.

Figure 2 shows serial HMPAO-SPECT studies obtained in two patients of similar age and with similar clinical symptomatology. Both patients were initially hemiplegic. In Case A a clear decrease of HMPAO uptake was detected 1 day after the insult in the left parietal and temporal region, which turned out to be 'hyperperfused' after 1 week. During this time period clinical symptomatology improved slightly, but still severe hemiparesis and moderate aphasia were present. The follow-up SPECT studies indicated the transition from hyperaemia to late oligaemia in the area of infarction, now also visible on CT. Neurological symptoms did not resolve completely in this patient. He was able to walk but hemiparesis and speech disturbance persisted and focal seizures evolving to generalized seizures appeared approximately 6 months after stroke occurrence.

At time of admission Case B suffered a progressive stroke. Initial hemiparesis deteriorated to hemiplegia. CT and Doppler sonography carried out within 2 h after admission, revealed normal brain tissue density (somewhat widened sulci were seen on CT) and patent neck vessels. By transcranial Doppler sonography no signal from the right middle cerebral artery could be detected, indicating a possible embolic occlusion of this vessel. Since the patient had a transplanted kidney, no angiography was performed. This first SPECT study obtained 1 day after the insult showed no circumscribed ischaemic lesion but there was some rightward asymmetry in hemispheric per cent-HMPAO uptake especially in the parietal and temporal region. Follow-up SPECT investigations revealed a slight decrease of this asymmetry, which was paralleled by an almost complete resolution of neurological symptoms after 5 weeks.

These two examples indicate the value of repeated follow-up CBF investigations. It can be assumed that the marked 'luxury perfusion' detected in Case A reflects an uncoupling between CBF and metabolism, which will lead to tissue necrosis and a persistent neurological deficit. We were able to observe in several stroke patients a similar time-related CBF pattern and all of them had suffered a completed stroke.

In contrast to the marked 'luxury perfusion' a mild, early increase of CBF, as shown in Case B, may reflect a favourable prognosis also in the presence of severe and long-lasting neurological disability. Probably such a CBF pattern indicates a reperfusion of an ischaemic brain within few hours, thus preventing it from a further drop of regional brain metabolism and ATP depletion, which would lead to neuronal death.

Vasomotor response may be detected by repeated SPECT investigations. Two approaches have been and are still used to estimate perfusion reserve in CVD patients. On the one hand vasoreactivity is tested after administration of acetazolamide or exposure to $CO_2$. There is no substantial difference between the two tests[46], although the mechanism of acetazolamide that leads to vasodilatation is not fully elucidated. The second approach is the combined detection of regional cerebral blood volume (rCBV) and CBF.

Acetazolamide induces in normal elderly controls according to Vorstrup et al.[58], a CBF increase of 31 per cent (13–46 per cent). The same authors used this test to investigate retrospectively the outcome of CVD patients after EC–IC bypass surgery. The best outcome had two out of 16 patients who preoperatively showed a distinct decrease of focal flow after acetazolamide ('steal effect'). Figure 3 indicates consecutive SPECT studies before and after EC–IC bypass surgery. In this single case perfusion reserve improved after surgery.

PET studies revealed a relationship between cerebral perfusion pressure, rCBV and rCBF[16]. In patients with severe uni- or bilateral carotid disease the perfusion drop is indicated by an increase

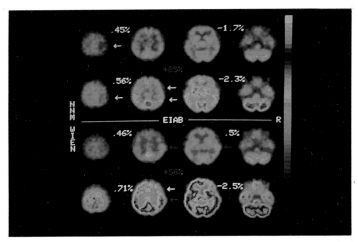

*Fig. 3. SPECT studies (images represent per cent HMPAO uptake/100 g) before and after i.v. adminis-tration of 1 g acetazolamide (ACA) obtained in a female patient, 50 years of age, who suffered a right cerebral RIND. Angiography revealed a 80 per cent stenosis of the right ICA. Left number columns dis-play global per cent HMPAO uptake, right columns the per cent left/right asymmetry. The baseline study (1st row) shows a decreased tracer uptake in the right parietal area (white arrow). After ACA (second row) this asymmetry became more prominent (white arrows) and global per cent HMPAO up-take increased by 25 per cent . After external–internal bypass surgery (3rd row) global per cent HMPAO uptake is essentially the same as in the baseline study, but left/right asymmetry decreased, due to a rCBF increase at the site of the anastomosis (red arrows). Global per cent HMPAO uptake after ACA (4th row) this time increased by 56 per cent, but a region of impaired vasomotor response in the right latero-frontal cortex (white arrow) is still visible.*

of rCBV due to vasodilation in the supply territory. The best discrimination between patent and occluded arterial territories was achieved by calculating the ratio rCBF/rCBV, since a critical rCBV could not be defined. This ratio is reciprocal to the mean vascular transit time and the lowest values were found in patients who had a haemodynamic rather than a thrombo-embolic cause of stroke. When vasodilatation is maximal any further decrease in perfusion pressure leads to a fall both in CBF and CBV. The brain compensates for this failure by increasing the oxygen extraction fraction (OEF) from the normal 40–50 per cent up to 85 per cent . Therefore a low rCBF/rCBV ratio reflects indirectly an increased OEF. Since red blood cells can be labelled with [99m]Tc, an rCBF/rCBV ratio can be calculated also by SPECT[9,32,56]. These authors were able to differentiate patient groups showing various stages of perfusion reserve.

Reduction of stroke incidence can be achieved by drug or surgical or combined treatment. For many years it has been known that aspirin has a preventive effect on stroke incidence. However, there are still debates on the effective inhibiting doses of platelet aggregation[27,55]. For the acute therapy of ischaemic stroke, calcium channel blockers such as nimodipine or haemodiluting agents are considered. The challenge to functional imaging would be a result-related selection of the appropriate therapeutic regimen for the individual patient. Although numerous exciting PET and SPECT studies in the field of CVD have been performed and knowledge of pathophysiologi-cal processes has thereby been increased, no definite strategy in the treatment of ischaemic stroke has been elaborated upon the basis of functional imaging results. PET studies gave some evi-dence of the positive influence on the outcome of stroke patients after oral nimodipine therapy[25]. However, a PET multitracer modality allowed to identify viable peri-infarct tissue up to 48 h after a stroke but progression to necrosis of this tissue could not be prevented by conventional therapeutic regimens[26]. The effect of surgical interventions[4,17,45] is still controversial. The major

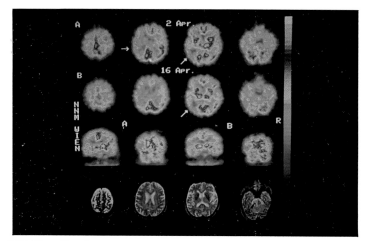

Fig. 4. Two SPECT studies (images represent per cent HMPAO uptake), 14 days apart, of a male patient, 60 years of age with initially plegic right arm, severe paresis and hypesthesia of the right leg. A mild motor aphasia could be observed. Clinically, a stroke in the territory of the left MCA was assumed. Surprisingly, MRI revealed a hyperintense (T2 weighted) area in the left pontine region, without any sign of supratentorial ischaemia (4th row, see arrow). The first SPECT study, performed on the 9th day after the insult showed a clear decrease of per cent HMPAO/100 g uptake in the left thalamus, to a lower degree in the left temporo-parietal region and in the latero-frontal cortex (arrows). The second SPECT study, 14 days later, revealed now a well-perfused thalamus but the left temporo-parietal region still showed a decreased tracer uptake. Per cent HMPAO uptake between the studies did not differ significantly, and average interhemispheric uptake difference was almost identical. The 3rd row displays coronal sections through the thalami and cerebellum. This finding indicates a deactivation of ponto-thalamic and thalamo-cortical connections. The patient improved during the following 3 weeks he was able to walk; but only with assistance due to a persistent hemiparesis. Impairment of sensibility in the right lower limb and motor aphasia cleared completely.

reason for this inconclusiveness is probably the high variability of the investigation time after the insult and different patient populations in the studies thus impeding significant statistical results. In the future well-designed studies are needed to estimate the optimal time window, drug therapy and the best surgical approach for selected patient groups.

Due to the complex connections between different brain areas, which are also partially unknown, remote effects in brain regions distant to the ischaemic lesion and caused by functional depression, can be studied. One of the best known is the so-called 'crossed cerebellar diaschisis'[3]. Fig. 4 shows the effect of pontine ischaemic lesion detected by repeated MRI studies, on rCBF in brain areas distant to the lesion. Clinically the patient presented the typical symptoms of a stroke in the territory supplied by the left middle cerebral artery (right hemiparesis and motor aphasia).

It can be summarized that in CVD, SPECT is useful for the recognition of rCBF impairment and its extent. Remote effects on primarily non-ischaemic brain tissue can be recorded. The prognosis for the restoration of neurological functions can be estimated based on repeated SPECT and CT (MRI) results, despite long-lasting severe neurological disability. However, SPECT or PET findings at present have no influence on the therapeutical regimen in cerebral ischaemia. Intracerebral and subarachnoidal haemorrhage – as it is known – is the diagnostic domain of CT. In this clinical condition SPECT can again be only of help in detecting deafferentation or the effect of vasospasm on rCBF.

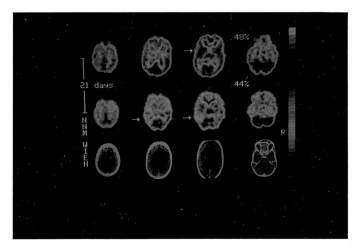

*Fig. 5. Two HMPAO-SPECT studies (separated by 21 days) obtained in a female patient 21 years of age who was treated for 2 years with various antidepressants because of mood disorders. No seizure history could be explored. On the day of the first SPECT investigation, she reported severe anxiety, restlessness, occasional short-lasting speech arrests and minimal jerks of the right thumb. The first SPECT study shows a slightly increased HMPAO uptake in the left insula (arrow, 1st row) suggesting partial seizures. The patient was treated with carbamazepine and the control SPECT study revealed a slight decrease of tracer deposition in the left temporal region (3rd row, arrows) while the patient was free of the symptoms above. CT scan was normal.*

### Epilepsy

Epilepsy is one of the neurological and psychiatric diseases which can manifest itself in the most bizarre way. Complaints are sometimes similar to neurasthenic, psychosomatic, hysteric or vegetative or even paranoid symptoms, so even experienced clinicians occasionally have difficulties in differentiating such states. Therefore, SPECT can have an important role for the differential diagnosis between seizures and 'seizure like' states (Fig. 5) in patients, where conventional EEG recordings are not conclusive.

It is well known that paroxysmal discharges are associated with increased local metabolism and blood flow in the brain tissue. A large number of investigations (two-dimensional $^{133}$Xe blood flow, PET and SPECT studies) were carried out during epileptic seizures or at different time intervals after a seizure[1,13,15,29,34,35,49]. Due to the different kinetics of the tracers applied in these investigations, the non-uniform usage of the terms 'interictal' and 'postictal', and the variability in spatial resolution of the used ECT-systems[50], the reported results in some of these studies can hardly be compared.

PET and SPECT investigations have shown that, in patients suffering from partial seizures, in approximately 60–86 per cent of the cases brain areas with impaired metabolism or CBF can be detected interictally[2,13,34,44], while subjects with generalized seizures usually have a normal regional metabolic or CBF pattern. Discordant results are most evident in cases where increased rCBF pattern was recorded even 2 weeks after the last clinically observable seizure[35], while in the EEG controlled postictal state (4–8 min after the seizure) an even more profound decrease in rCBF than in the interictal state was found by Rowe *et al.*[49]. Since the tracer HMPAO was used in these studies, tracer kinetics can not explain the divergence. Hougaard *et al.*[29] have also detected, with $^{133}$Xe, increased rCBF in epileptic patients despite normal scalp EEG and absence

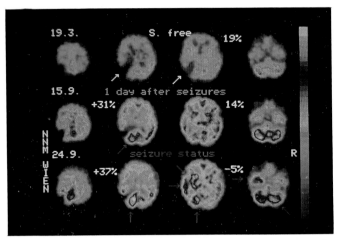

*Fig. 6. SPECT study (1st rwo) in the interictal state of a female patient 47 years of age who developed partial complex seizures aftger a left parietal angioma was removed by operation. The 2nd row displays the SPECT investigation after a seizure status. An increased HMPAO deposition is visible in the left sup. occipital region at the border of the left parietal structural lesion. During a seizure status (3rd row) the increased HMPAO uptake extends from the occipital to the temporal lobe and to the anterior basal ganglia on the left. During the seizures the patient had optical hallucinations.*

of seizures. Besides the case reported by Lang *et al.*[35], we and others (Deisenhammer *et al.*, 1993, personal communication) have observed in several instances a long lasting increase of HMPAO deposition after a seizure. The location of the maximally increased HMPAO deposition was also slightly changing thus suggesting migration of the epileptogenic zone (Fig. 6). Obviously, in these patients there was no evidence of underlying encephalitis, which would have as a consequence a persistent regional HMPAO accumulation. In our opinion, prolonged postictal regional tracer accumulation is dependent on the frequency of seizures preceding the postictal SPECT since all the observed cases had frequent seizures or an epileptic status.

Reports on the beneficial effect of surgery in patients with medically refractory partial seizures of temporal lobe origin are available today[12]. The detection of the epileptogenic tissue is sometimes difficult and several techniques are applied in specialized centres in order to identify the brain area responsible for seizure onset. Extracranial EEG coupled with long-term intensive monitoring, recordings from sphenoidal electrodes, MRI and ECT are predominantly used. In cases where these techniques give congruent results, there is no need for further invasive investigation with stereotactically implanted intracranial depth electrodes. With increasing spatial resolution of MRI and ECT atrophic changes, small tumours and functionally impaired brain tissue in the hippocampal region can be detected with higher accuracy. Engel and co-workers[14] reported an increase of positive PET studies in candidates for surgery up to 86 per cent by using a high resolution scanner. Thus PET and SPECT play an important role in defining epileptogenic tissue. It is desirable to have an on-site opportunity of EEG recording and tracer injection in order to relate perfusion abnormalities to EEG findings with greater accuracy. In our opinion focus detection is also enhanced by comparison of ictal and interictal SPECT (PET). A further approach to improve the contrast between normal and pathological brain tissue is the use of associative automatic speech as stimulus which leads to an increase of brain metabolism (or CBF) in normal tissue (Pawlik & Heiss, in preparation). PET and SPECT can also help to determine where to place subdural grid or strip electrodes in patients with extratemporal seizures.

From the above mentioned, it is clear that ECT results have a practical impact on the management and therapeutic strategy of seizure patients.

### Dementias

Dementias are a heterogeneous group of diseases, which have in common a clinical pattern of acquired, global and progressive impairment of intellectual performance, loss of memory and personality disturbance, exceeding similar features occurring during normal ageing. The classification of dementias into cortical and subcortical seems to be unfortunate since all of them are characterized by degenerative processes that involve cortical and subcortical brain regions during progression of the disease. Of more practical clinical importance is the differentiation between Alzheimer's disease and multi-infarct dementia (MID) or subcortical encephalopathy (Binswanger's disease) because of the dramatic differences in patient management. Whilst the progression of multi-infarct can be delayed by the use of vasoactive drugs, there is no benefit for patients with dementia of the Alzeheimer type (DAT) from drug therapy, at the moment. However, the definition of characteristic patterns of brain perfusion for each of the different dementias will help the identification of pure samples of MID and DAT to be enrolled in drug efficacy trials. Alzheimer's disease (45–60 per cent of the dementias) shows, according to several studies, a more or less characteristic distribution pattern of rCBF or glucose metabolism[22,24,30,41]. Fig. 7 indicates the typical findings of advanced DAT with a marked bilateral decrease of rCBF in the temporal, parietal and frontal cortex, while the motor and the visual cortices as well as the subcortical structures are relatively well perfused. However, in early stages of the disease, the appearances are different. The disease involves primarily the temporal and parietal cortices and progresses to the frontal cortex at later stages. Repeat SPECT investigations, separated by 4–6 months, may show a distinct progression of neuronal loss, matching the described necropsic observations regarding distribution of plaques of amyloid. Multi-infarct dementia (15–25 per cent of the dementias) as well as subcortical encephalopathy can be recognized by the combination of CT (or MRI) and SPECT (or PET) investigations[11]. Both types of studies reveal ischaemic lesions with clearly lowered HMPAO uptake (SPECT) in the white matter and/or atrophic cortical changes. It has to be pointed out that it is essential to compare the results of

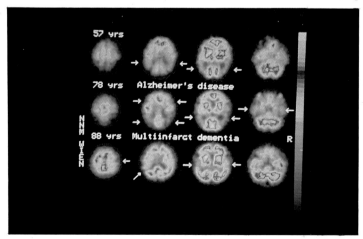

*Fig. 7. The 1st row displays a typical SPECT finding in presumed Alzheimer's disease (female patient, 57 years of age). HMPAO deposition is markedly decreased in the parietal and temporal lobe on either sides (arrows). The same SPECT finding is obtained in senile dementia of the Alzheimer type (female patient, 78 years of age). Row 3 shows a SPECT finding in multi-infarct dementia (male patient, 88 years of age).*

morphological and functional brain imaging in order to obtain improved accuracy in the diagnosis of dementia.

Pathological SPECT or PET findings can be also found in the early stages of Huntington's disease[6,20,23], when atrophy of the caudate nucleus is not detected with CT or MRI. Pick's disease, also called dementia of the frontal lobe type, has been associated with a marked decrease of regional brain perfusion and metabolism in the frontal cortex, sometimes involving the cortex of temporal lobes[24,31]. Although not specific, abnormalities of brain perfusion and chemistry (metabolism of glucose) found in several degenerative disorders of the central nervous system may be detected with SPECT and PET. For instance, there have been sporadic reports demonstrating these abnormalities in patients with AIDS-dementia complex[57], mitochondrial encephalomyopathy[21], Creutzfeld–Jacob disease[54] and supranuclear palsy[18,37]. In the latter, more specific findings can be expected from $D_2$-dopamine receptor SPECT studies as it is mentioned below. Interestingly another pathological condition of difficult diagnosis and poor outcome, herpes virus encephalitis, has benefited from brain perfusion SPECT finding. In the early phase of the disease (first week) there is circumscribed focal increase of the brain perfusion tracer uptake in the mesial cortex of one of the temporal lobes, which becomes photodeficient on the later stages (more than 1 month) of the viral encephalitis[28,52]. SPECT or PET are also very important diagnostic tools for the differentiation between truly demented states and pseudo-dementia caused by severe depression. Reduced rCBF is usually confined to the frontal lobes (more pronounced on the left). Other cortical areas may show almost normal rCBF distribution. Repeat studies post-therapy are imperative to demonstrate improvement of the regional perfusion pattern to the frontal cortex and to establish the differential diagnosis – depression *vs* dementia.

Finally, quantitative SPECT or PET permit a more objective evaluation of the effects of a certain therapeutic regimen. The combination of SPECT data with fine neuropsychological testing increases the diagnostic accuracy in dementia[19].

### *Head trauma*

It is difficult to understand the present role of brain perfusion SPECT and metabolic PET studies in the evaluation of late effects of post-traumatic personality and intellectual changes. Debate about the potential of 'functional brain imaging' as a legal proof of an individual social abnormal behaviour will continue for some time to come. However, there are already some studies demonstrating that CBF studies reveal more abnormalities than CT or MRI[42,48]. The potential predictive value of brain perfusion SPECT to define the outcome of patients with intracranial post-traumatic haematomas reported in the literature[10] needs further evaluation in larger samples.

### *Brain death*

The potential application of brain perfusion tracers in the confirmation of irreversible brain damage is based on the fact that lack of uptake and retention of those tracers in the brain reflects severe neuronal loss. The methodology is simple and can be carried out at the bedside once planar images are taken frequently enough to demonstrate the lack of tracer uptake. In cases of doubt, particularly of brain stem death, SPECT may be a useful addition. There have been several reports in the literature demonstrating the high accuracy of this method which has shown no false positives[47,51].

### Receptor studies

With SPECT at present, only $D_2$-dopamine receptors can be visualized with a relatively good spatial resolution. Benzamide derivatives such as raclopride (used for $D_2$ dopamine receptor PET studies) or iodobenzamide (IBZM, used for SPECT) have a high affinity to $D_2$ dopamine recep-

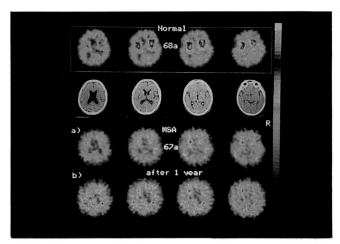

*Fig. 8. The 1st row displays the IBZM SPECT study of a normal control subject for comparison with the IBZM SPECT findings in a 67-year-old female patient suffering from multisystem atrophy (MSA). Initially (a) little tracer binding is visible in the striatum while with disease progression after 1 year (b) only unspecific IBZM binding can be detected. The normal CT scan of the patient is shown in row 2.*

tors. Recently new receptor subclasses have been discovered. $D_3$ and $D_4$ receptors have some pharmacological similarity to the $D_2$ receptor but are preponderantly located in limbic and cortical areas of the brain. However, the density of $D_2$ dopamine receptors in the striatum is much higher than those of $D_3$ and $D_4$ receptors and therefore the amount of IBZM bound to these receptors is negligible.

In several studies[7,8] it was shown that with this compound PET results could be replicated in larger patient populations. A significant decrease of $D_2$ dopamine receptors with age ($r = 0.77$, $P < 0.001$) was found in normals but also to a lesser extent ($r = 0.43$, $P < 0.01$) in patients with Parkinson's disease (PD). An interesting finding in PD was the absence of a significant correlation between receptor binding and duration of the disease, or severity of clinical symptoms of L-dopa treatment.

Of practical clinical value is the differentiation between PD and multisystem atrophy or progressive supranuclear palsy (Steele–Richardson–Olszewsky syndrome). While in PD the striatal/frontal cortex ratio is within the normal range, in the other two degenerative disorders this ratio is clearly reduced (Fig. 8). IBZM-SPECT is further useful in the diagnosis of Huntington's disease, in which a profound decrease of $D_2$ dopamine receptor density can also be found in the early stages of the disease. It was a clinical observation that chronic treatment of CVD or migraine patients with cinnarizine and flunarize can cause depressive symptoms. According to new results (Brücke & Wöber, in preparation) these drugs are blocking $D_2$ dopamine receptors to some extent and can cause a deterioration of extrapyramidal symptoms. This is a classical example for therapeutic decision making based on the recognition of – in this case negative – drug effects by functional imaging. In psychiatry the $D_2$ dopamine receptor blockade by 'classical' neuroleptics (which can cause dose-dependent, severe extrapyramidal symptoms as a side effect) can be detected and antipsychotic drugs can be classified according to their blocking potency.

Benzodiazepine receptors can also be visualized with iomazenil-SPECT. This compound was used for the detection of epileptogenic foci. Results obtained in a multicentre study[53] did not reveal a clear-cut advantage of iomazenil over HMPAO in the visual detection of brain areas with impaired function. Since benzodiazepine receptors are located in the whole cortex and to a lesser extent in subcortical structures or white matter, tracer distribution ratios representing abnormal receptor density can hardly be calculated – in contrast to $D_2$ dopamine receptors, where a high signal difference exists between cortex and striatum. Therefore at present, iomazenil SPECT is not of great importance in neurological nuclear medicine. However, the new SPECT systems, which allow fast rotation of detectors and consequently dynamic tracer inflow studies, will probably make quantification of receptor densities possible. If any differences in benzodiazepine receptor density exist in the various forms of epilepsy, such a procedure will allow their detection in the future.

## References

1. Abou-Khalil, B.W., Siegel, G.J., Sackellares, J.C., Gilman, S., Hichwa, R. & Marshall, R. (1987): Positron emission tomography studies of cerebral glucose metabolism in chronic partial epilepsy. *Ann. Neurol.* **22**, 480–486.

2. Andersen, A.R., Waldemar, G., Dam, M., Fuglsang-Frederiksen, A., Herning, M., Kruse–Larsen, C. & Lassen, N.A. (1990): SPECT and EEG in focal epilepsy with and without normal CT and MRI scans – a preliminary study in 28 cases. In: *Current problems in epilepsy*, eds. M. Baldy-Moulinier, N.A. Lassen, J. Engel Jr., S. Askienazy, pp. 97–104. London, Paris, Rome: John Libbey.

3. Baron, J.C., Bousser, M.G., Comar, D. & Castaigne, P. (1980): 'Crossed cerebellar diaschisis' in human supratentorial brain infarction. *Trans. Am. Neurol. Assoc.* **105**, 459–461.

4. Baron, J.C., Bousser, M.G., Rey, A., Guillard, A., Comar, D. & Castaigne, P. (1981): Reversal of focal 'misery-perfusion syndrome' by extra-intracranial arterial bypass in hemodynamic cerebral ischaemia. *Stroke* **12**, 454–459.

5. Baron, J.C. (1987): Ischaemic stroke studied by 150-labelled compounds: misery perfusion and luxury perfusion. In: *Clinical efficacy of positron emission tomography*, eds. W.-D. Heiss, G. Pawlik, K. Herholz, K. Wienhard, pp. 15–23. Dodrecht: Martinus Nijhoff.

6. Berent, S., Giordani, B., Lehtinen, S., Markel, D., Penny, J.B., Buchtel, H.A., Starosta-Rubinstein, S., Hichwa, R. & Young, A.B. (1988): Positron emission tomography scan investigations of Huntington's disease: cerebral metabolic correlates of cognitive function. *Ann. Neurol.* **23**, 541–546.

7. Brücke, T., Podreka, I., Angelberger, P., Wenger, S., Topitz, A., Küfferle, B., Müller, Ch. & Deecke, L. (1991): Dopamine D2 receptor imaging with SPECT. Studies in different neuropsychiatric disorders. *J. Cereb. Blood Flow Metab.* **11**, 220–228.

8. Brücke, T., Podreka, I., Wenger, S., Angelberger, P., Müller, Ch., Walter, H., Strobl, R. & Deecke, L. (1991): Dopamine receptor imaging with SPECT: a diagnostic tool in extrapyramidal disorders and *in vivo* assay for the measurement of receptor blockade by neuroleptic treatment. *J. Cereb. Blood Flow Metab.* **11** (S2), S877.

9. Buell, U., Braun, H., Ferbert, A., Stirner, H., Weiller, C. & Ringelstein, E.B. (1988): Combined SPECT imaging of regional cerebral blood flow ($^{99m}$Tc-hexamethyl-propyleneamine oxime, HMPAO) and blood volume ($^{99m}$Tc-RBC) to assess regional cerebral perfusion reserve in patients with cerebrovascular disease. *NuklearMedizin* **27**, 51–56.

10. Choksey, M.S., Costa, D.C., Iannotti, F., Ell, P.J. & Crockard, H.A. (1991): $^{99m}$Tc-HMPAO SPECT studies in traumatic intracerebral haematoma. *J. Neurol. Neurosurg. Psychiatry*, **54**, 6–11.

11. De Chiara, S., Lassen, N.A., Andersen, A.R., Gade, A., Lester, J., Thomsen, C. & Henriksen, O. (1987): High-resolution nuclear magnetic resonance imaging and single photon emission computerized tomography – cerebral blood flow in a case of pure sensory stroke and mild dementia owing to subcortical arteriosclerotic encephalopathy (Binswanger's disease). *Am. J. Physiol. Imag.* **2**, 192–195.

12. Delgado-Escueta, A.V. & Walsh, G.O. (1985): Type I complex partial seizures of hippocampal origin: excellent results of anterior temporal lobectomy. *Neurology* **35**, 143–154.

13. Engel, J.Jr., Kuhl, D.E. & Phelps M.E. (1982): Patterns of human local cerebral glucose metabolism during epileptic seizures. *Science* **218**, 64–66.

14. Engel, J.Jr., Henry, T.R., Risinger, M.W., Mazziotta, J.C., Sutherling, W.W., Levesque, M.F. & Phelps, M.E. (1990): Presurgical evaluation for partial epilepsy: relative contributions of chronic depth-electrode recordings *vs* FDG-PET and scalp-sphenoidal ictal EEG. *Neurology* **40**, 1670–1677.

15. Feindel, W., Yamamoto, L., Thompson, C. & Matsunaga, M. (1980): Positron emission tomography for cerebral blood flow measurement and detection of focal lesions in epilepsy. In: *Advances in epileptology*, XIth Epilepsy International Symposium, eds. R. Canger, P. Angeleri & J.K. Penry, pp. 73–81. New York: Raven Press.

16. Gibbs, J.M., Wise, R.J.S., Leenders, K.L. & Jones, T. (1984): Evaluation of cerebral perfusion reserve in patients with carotid artery occlusion. *Lancet* **i**, 310–314.

17. Gibbs, J.M., Wise R.J.S., Thomas, D.J., Mansfield, A.O. & Ross Russel, R.W. (1989): Cerebral hemodynamic changes after extracranial–intracranial bypass surgery. *J. Neurol. Neurosurg. Psychiatry* **50**, 140–150.

18. Goffinet, A.M., De Volder, A.G., Gillian, C., Rectem, D., Bol, A., Michel, C., Cogneau, M., Labar, D. & Laterre, C. (1989): Positron tomography demonstrates frontal lobe hypometabolism in progressive supranuclear palsy. *Ann. Neurol.* **25**, 131–139.

19. Goldenberg, G., Podreka, I., Suess, E. & Deecke, L. (1989): The cerebral localisation of neuropsychological impairment in Alzheimer's disease. *J. Neurol.* **236**, 131–138.

20. Grafton, S.T., Mazziotta, J.C., Pahl, J.J., St. George-Hyslop, P., Haines, J.L., Gusella, J., Hoffman, J.M., Baxter, L.R. & Phelps, M.E. (1990): A comparison of neurological, metabolic, structural, and genetic evaluations in persons at risk for Huntington's disease. *Ann. Neurol.* **28**, 614–621.

21. Grünwald, F., Zierz, S., Broich, K., Schumacher, S., Bockisch, A. & Biersack, H. (1990): HMPAO-SPECT imaging resembling Alzheimer-type dementia in mitochondrial encephalomyopathy with lactic acidosis and stroke-like episodes (MELAS). *J. Nucl. Med.* **31**, 1740–1742.

22. Haxby, J.V., Duara, R., Grady, C.L., Cutler, N.R. & Rapoport, S.I. (1985): Relations between neuropsychological and cerebral metabolic asymmetries in early Alzheimer's disease. *J. Cereb. Blood Flow Metab.* **5**, 193–200.

23. Hayden, M.R., Martin, W.R.W., Stoessl, A.J., Clark, C., Hollenberg, S., Adam, M.J., Ammann, W., Harrop, R., Rogers, J., Ruth, T., Sayre, C. & Pate, B.D. (1986): Positron emission tomography in the early diagnosis of Huntington's disease. *Neurology* **36**, 888–894.

24. Heiss, W.D., Herholz, K., Pawlik, G. & Szelies, B. (1988): Beitrag der Positronen-Emissions-Tomographie zur Diagnose der Demenz. *Dtsch. Med. Wschr.* **113**, 1362–1367.

25. Heiss, W.D., Holthoff, V., Pawlik, G. & Neveling, M. (1990): Effect of Nimodipine on regional cerebral glucose metabolism in patients with acute ischaemic stroke as measured by positron emission tomography. *J. Cereb. Blood Flow Metab.* **10**, 127–132.

26. Heiss, W.D., Huber, M., Fink, G.R., Herholz, K., Pietrzyk, U., Wagner, R. & Wienhard, K. (1992): Progressive derangement of peri-infarct viable tissue in ischaemic stroke. *J. Cereb. Blood Flow Metab.* **12**, 193–203.

27. Helgason, C.M., Tortorice, K.L., Winkler, S.R., Penney, D.W., Schuler, J.J., McClelland, T.J. & Brace, L.D. (1983): Aspirin response and failure in cerebral infarction. *Stroke* **24**, 345–350.

28. Henkes, H., Huber, C., Hierholzer, J., Jaeger, H., Hammann, G. & Piepgras, U. (1991): Temporal-medial hot spot in HMPAO/SPET: key finding in acute herpes encephalitis. *Radiology* **18**,(P): 173.

29. Hougaard, K., Oikawa, T., Sveinsdottir, E., Skinhøj, E., Ingvar, D.H. & Lassen, N.A. (1976): Regional cerebral blood flow in focal cortical epilepsy. *Arch. Neurol.* **33**, 527–535.

30. Jagust, W.J., Budinger, T.F. & Redd, B.R. (1987): The diagnosis of dementia with single photon emission computed tomography. *Arch. Neurol.* **44**, 258–262.

31. Kamo, H., McGeer, P.L., Harrop, R., McGeer, E.G., Calne, D.B., Martin, W.R.W. & Pate, B.D. (1987): Positron emission tomography and histopathology in Pick's disease. *Neurology* **37**, 439–445.

32. Knapp, W., Von Kummer, R. & Kübler, W. (1986): Imaging of cerebral blood flow to volume distribution using SPECT. *J. Nucl. Med.* **27**, 465–470.

33. Kuhl, D.E., Phelps, M.E., Kowel, I.A.P., Metter, E.J., Selin, C. & Winter, J. (1980): Effects of stroke on local cerebral metabolism and perfusion: mapping by emission computed tomography of $^{18}$FDG and $^{13}$NH$_3$. *Ann. Neurol.* **8**, 47–60.

34. Kuhl, D.E., Engel, J.Jr. & Phelps, M.E. (1981): Emission computed tomography of $^{18}$FDG and $^{13}$NH$_3$ in partial epilepsy. In: *Cerebrovascular disease*, eds. J. Mossy & O.M. Reinmuth, pp. 73–75. New York: Raven Press.

35. Lang, W., Podreka, I., Suess, E., Müller, Ch., Zeitlhofer, J. & Deecke, L. (1988): Single photon emission computed tomography during and between seizures. *J. Neurol.* **235**, 277–284.

36. Lassen, N.A. (1966): The luxury-perfusion syndrome and its possible relation to acute metabolic acidosis localized within the brain. *Lancet* **ii**, 1113–1115.

37. Leenders, K.L., Frackowiak, R.S.J. & Lees, A.J. (1988): Steele–Richardson–Olszewski syndrome. Brain energy metabolism, blood flow and flourodopa uptake measured by positron emission tomography. *Brain* **111**, 615–630.

38. Matsuda, H., Tsuji, S., Shuke, N., Sumiya, H., Kuji, E. & Hisada, K. (1993): Noninvasive regional cerebral blood flow measurements using technetium-99m hexamethylpropylene amine oxime. *J. Nucl. Med.* **34**, 92P.

39. Matsuda, H., Tsuji, S., Shuke, N., Sumiya, H., Tonami, N. & Hisada, K. (1992): A quantitative approach to technetium-99m hexamethylpropylene amine oxime ($^{99m}$Tc-HMPAO). *Eur. J. Nucl. Med.* **19**, 195–200.

40. Mazziotta, J.C., Phelps, M.E., Miller, J. & Kuhl, D.E. (1981): Tomographic mapping of human cerebral metabolism: normal unstimulated state. *Neurology* **31**, 503–516.

41. Neary, D., Snowden, J.S., Shields, R.A., Burjan, A.W.I., Northern, B., MacDermot, N., Prescott, M.C. & Testa, H.J. (1987): Single photon emission tomography using $^{99m}$Tc-HMPAO in the investigation of dementia. *J. Neurol. Neurosurg. Psychiatry* **50**, 1101–1109.

42. Newton, M.R., Greenwood, R.J., Briton, K.E., Charlesworth, M., Nimmon, C.C., Carroll, M.J. & Dolke, G. (1992): A study comparing SPECT with CT and MRI after closed head injury. *J. Neurol. Neurosurg. Psychiatry.* **55**, 92–94.

43. Podreka, I., Asenbaum, S., Brücke, T., Wenger, S., Lang, W., Goldenberg, G., Schmidbauer, M. & Deecke, L. (1991): Intra-individual reproducibility of HMPAO brain uptake. *J. Cereb. Blood Flow Metab.* (Suppl. 2), S776.

44. Podreka, I., Lang, W., Suess, E., Wimberger, D., Steiner, M., Gradner, W., Zeithlhofer, J., Pelzl, G., Mamoli, B. & Deecke, L. (1988): Hexa-methyl-propylene-amine-oxime (HMPAO) single photon emission computed tomography (SPECT) in epilepsy. *Brain Topography* **1**, 55–60.

45. Powers, J.W., Press, G.A., Grubb, R.L., Gado, M. & Raichle, M.E. (1987): The effect of hemodynamically significant carotid artery disease on the hemodynamic status of the cerebral circulation. *Ann. Intern. Med.* **106**, 27–35.

46. Ringelstein, E.B., Van Eyck, S. & Mertens, I. (1992): Evaluation of cerebral vasomotor reactivity by various vasodilating stimuli: comparison of $CO_2$ to acetazolamide. *J. Cereb. Blood Flow Metab.* **12**, 162–168.

47. Riva, A., Gonzales, F.M., LLamas-Elvira, J.M., Latre, J.M., Jimenez-Hefferman, A., Vidal, E., Martinez, M., Torres, M., Guerrero, R., Alvarez, F. & Mateo, A. (1992): A diagnosis of brain death: superiority of perfusion studies with $^{99m}$Tc-HMPAO over convential radionuclide cerebral angiography. *Br. J. Radiol.* **65**, 289–294.

48. Roper, S.N., Mena, I., King, W.A., Schweitzer, J., Garrett, K., Mehringer, C.M. & McBride, D. (1991): An analysis of cerebral blood flow in acute closed-head injury using technetium-99m-HMPAO SPECT and computed tomography. *J. Nucl. Med.* **32**, 1684–1687.

49. Rowe, C.C., Berkovic, S.F., Austin, M.C., McKay, W.J. & Bladin, P.F. (1991): Patterns of postictal cerebral blood flow in temporal lobe epilepsy. *Neurology* **41**, 1096–1103.

50. Ryvlin, P., Phillipon, B., Cinotti, L., Froment, J.C., Le Bars, D. & Mauguiere, F. (1992): Functional neuroimaging strategy in temporal lobe epilepsy: a comparative study of $^{18}$FDG-PET and $^{99m}$Tc-HMPAO-SPECT. *Ann. Neurol.* **31**, 650–656.

51. Schlake, H.-P., Bëottger, I.G., Grotmeyer, K.-H., Husstedt, I.W., Brandau, W. & Schober, O. (1992): Determination of cerebral perfusion by means of planar scintigraphy and $^{99m}$Tc-HMPAO in brain death, persistent vegetative state and severe coma. *Intensive Care Med.* **18**, 76–81.

52. Schmidbauer, M., Podreka, I., Wimberger, D., Oder W., Koch, G., Wenger, S., Goldenberg, G., Asenbaum, S. & Deecke, L. (1991): SPECT and MRI imaging in herpes simplex encephalitis. *J. Comp. Assist. Tomogr.* **15**, 812–815.

53. Schubiger, P.A., Hasler, P.H., Beer-Wohlfahrt, H., Bekier, A., Oettli, R., Cordes, M., Ferstl, F., Deisenhammer, E., De Roo, M., Moser, E., Nitzsche, E., Podreka, I., Riccabona, G., Bangerl, I., Schober, O., Bartenstein, P., Van Rijk, P., Van Isselt, J.W., Van Royen, E.A., Verhoeff, N.P.L.G., Haldemann, R. & Von Schulthess, G.K. (1991): Evaluation of a multicentre study with iomazenil – a benzodiazepine receptor ligand. *Nucl. Med. Commun.* **12**, 569–582.

54. Shih, W.J., Markesbery, W.R., Clark, D.B., Goldstein, S., Domstad, P.A., Coupal, J.J., Kung, H., DeKosky, S.T. & Deland, F.H. (1987): I-123 HIPDM brain imaging findings in subacute spongiform encephalopathy (Creutzfeldt–Jacob disease). *J. Nucl. Med.* **28**, 1484–1487.

55. The Dutch TIA Study Group (1991): A comparison of two doses of aspirin (30 mg *vs* 283 mg a day) in patients after a transient ischaemic attack or minor ischaemic stroke. *N. Engl. J. Med.* **325**, 1261–1266.

56. Toyama, H., Takeshita, G., Takeuchi, A., Anno, H., Ejiri, K., Maeda, H., Katada, K., Koga, S., Ishijama, N., Kanno, T. & Yamaoka, N. (1990): Cerebral hemodynamics in patients with chronic obstructive carotid disease by rCBF, rCBV, and rCBV/rCBF ratio using SPECT. *J. Nucl. Med.* **31,** 55–60.

57. Tran Dinh, Y.R., Mamo, H., Cervoni, J., Caulin, C. & Saimot, A.C. (1990): Disturbances in the cerebral perfusion of human immune deficiency virus-1 seropositive asymptomatic subjects: a quantitative tomography study of 18 cases. *J. Nucl. Med.* **31,** 1601–1607.

58. Vorstrup, S., Brun, B. & Lassen, N.A. (1986): Evaluation of the cerebral vasodilatory capacity by the acetazolamide test before EC–IC bypass surgery in patients with occlusion of the internal carotid artery. *Stroke* **17,** 1291–1298.

*New Trends in Nuclear Neurology and Psychiatry*, edited by D.C. Costa, G.F. Morgan and N. A. Lassen
© 1993 John Libbey & Company Ltd., pp. 119–131

# Chapter 8

# Brain SPET in neuropsychiatry – activation studies in health and disease

Howard Ring

*Lecturer in Neuropsychiatry, Institute of Neurology, Queen Square, London WC1*

## Introduction

There is a long-held belief that our understanding of the cerebral basis of behaviours will be advanced by attempts to localize behaviours to specific brain regions. This approach has had mixed success. The phrenologists of the 18th century attempted to understand features of personality in terms of the variable sizes of hypothetical cerebral organs each supposedly subserving highly specialized behavioural functions. Whilst this particular theory was distinctly unsuccessful, the careful clinical observations by Broca of the effects of a localized lesion on the articulation of speech set the scene for a productive approach that has indeed contributed to our understanding of the cerebral basis of language.

Lesion studies have advanced enormously our appreciation of mechanisms of cerebral function but, as pointed out by Hughlings Jackson and re-emphasized by Luria[41], the consequences of a cerebral lesion reveal not the function of the damaged area but the capabilities of the intact portions of the brain. In addition, inferences of brain function drawn from lesion studies are vulnerable to the confounding effects of inaccuracies in defining the extent of neuronal damage, and assumptions both of a local loss of neuronal function in the damaged area and of unaffected activity in cerebral sites distant to the lesion.

## Functional neuroimaging: relevance for neuropsychiatry

With the advent of functional neuroimaging it has for the first time become possible to examine tomographically localized spatially distributed ongoing activity in the intact brain. These techniques may be particularly valuable in the study of neuropsychiatric states, a possible definition of which will be attempted. In part, neuropsychiatry is the study and management of the psychological and psychiatric sequelae of demonstrable cerebral pathology (for instance depression and psychoses developing in patients with epilepsy, Parkinson's disease or a dementing illness). However, the term also describes a particular approach to investigating what may be thought of as primary psychiatric disorders (for instance schizophrenia or obsessive compulsive disorder), based on examination of cerebral, as opposed perhaps to psychosocial, functioning. The aim of neuropsychiatric investigation is to explore the nature of biological links between specific cerebral regions or processes and aspects of psychopathology. Structural imaging techniques have been of great value in the elucidation of neurological diseases with well-defined pathology. However, they have not produced clear evidence towards the basis of even a single human psychopathological state. It is reasonable to take the optimistic view that since psychopathological disturbances are by definition disturbances of function, rather than of structure, then the detailed imaging of cerebral function may be more revealing in these circumstances than structural investigations.

Cerebral activity may be observed whilst subjects are at rest or during the performance of mental work, as well as in association with pharmacological challenges, in both healthy and dysfunctional brains. Measurement of regional cerebral blood flow (rCBF) has been described as the most accurate signal of changes in local neuronal activity that can be detected by current functional neuroimaging techniques[19,57]. In this chapter both resting state studies and findings from blood flow measurements obtained during the performance of various tasks will be discussed.

### Resting state studies

SPET studies have contributed both to clinical management of and research into a variety of neuropsychiatric states. Two studies have investigated the phenomenon of transient global amnesia. This uncommon condition is poorly understood but has been associated with cerebrovascular disease. It is also of interest as a paradigm to investigate the neural basis of memory. The phenomenon itself refers to a brief and fully reversible but complete anterograde amnesia with limited retrograde amnesia. SPET blood flow scans during the episode have demonstrated widespread cerebral hypoperfusion, with particular decreases in medial temporal structures and the thalami[24,61]. As well as providing a valuable insight into some of the cerebral mechanisms of memory, the results demonstrate a value for SPET in aiding the differential diagnosis between transient global amnesia and the psychiatric condition of a dissociative hysterical state, which is not known to be associated with any specific perfusion deficits.

Resting state blood flow studies have been valuable in helping to define the cerebral correlates of distinct syndromes of cognitive decline. The bilateral temporal and posterior parietal hypoperfusion of Alzheimer's dementia is well recognized[10]. This pattern has been compared to the results obtained from other dementing processes in an attempt to understand whether similar pathological processes may operate. Idiopathic Parkinson's disease is a common condition. In the United States 1 per cent of the population over 50 years of age is known to be affected[1]. It has been estimated that 15 per cent of these patients will develop generalized cognitive decline[9,64]. However, it has not been clear whether this is a dementing process specific to IPD or whether it is a form of Alzheimer type dementia. In a study of 15 patients with IPD and dementia, 15 patients with IPD alone, 19 patients with Alzheimer's dementia and 13 control subjects, regional cortical to cerebellar ratios in non-demented IPD patients did not differ from the controls. However, the two groups with dementia shared a common pattern of hypoperfusion predominant in parieto-temporal cortices, although the perfusion deficits were greater in the Alzheimer group[60]. The authors conclude that their results support the conclusion that dementia in IPD may be due to the coexistence of IPD and Alzheimer's dementia.

Although it is still generally accepted that the explanation for the development of dementia in IPD has yet to be firmly established, this example demonstrates the value that SPET imaging has in furthering understanding the cerebral basis of cognitive and behavioural pathologies. Similarly, resting state $^{99m}$Tc-HMPAO have been used to distinguish patterns of cerebral perfusion associated with Alzheimer's dementia and another condition characterized by severe memory deficits: Korsakoff's psychosis[31]. In this case, where pathological studies have indicated quite different cerebral lesions in the two conditions, the SPET results were likewise different. The patients with the latter condition demonstrated preserved posterior temporal perfusion but impaired frontal lobe perfusion. This frontal hypoperfusion was significantly correlated with performance on psychological tests sensitive to frontal lobe integrity.

Other primary degenerative dementias have also been distinguished with the aid of SPET characterization. Neary and colleagues[49,50] have described a frontal lobe dementing syndrome with associated cognitive and behavioral disturbances. They used SPET scan results from these patients, all of whom demonstrated selective reductions of tracer uptake in the anterior cerebral hemispheres, to confirm the association between the observed clinical phenomena and frontal lobe dysfunction. In another study of patients with frontal lobe dementia it was demonstrated that in six of the eight patients examined, magnetic resonance imaging failed to localize frontal dysfunction that was observed clinically and with SPET[48].

Biological investigations into possible cerebral associations of what are generally considered as primary psychiatric diseases have until recently been limited to structural imaging and the use of neuroendocrine challenges. Neither of these approaches has been particularly successful. Hence the introduction of functional imaging of psychiatric states has been greeted with much enthusiasm. Although no specific answers have yet been provided, there is at least a consensus emerging from positron emission tomography (PET) and SPET investigations particularly of depression and obsessive compulsive disorder (OCD). Measures of both regional cerebral blood flow and local glucose metabolic rates have demonstrated left hemisphere medial prefrontal cortical hypoactivity in depression[4-7]. Baxter and colleagues also found a normalization of this focal hypoactivity following antidepressant medication. Interestingly, in depression occurring in patients with idiopathic Parkinson's disease and with which it appears to have a particular association, a PET study of regional glucose metabolism also demonstrated hypometabolism within the prefrontal cortex, in this case in the orbital-inferior area[44]. The convergence of these findings from similar behavioural states associated with differing diseases, provides supportive evidence for a central role for the prefrontal cortex in the mediation of depressive states.

In the case of OCD the findings have been even more promising. In part this may be because OCD appears to be one of the very few pathological states (ictal epilepsy is another) in which pathology appears to be specifically related to focal hyperactivity, rather than to hypoactivity which as a function of its frequent occurrence in conditions as varied as depression, autism, schizophrenia, chronic alcoholism and coma is a less specific finding[18,42,63]. The hyperactivity of OCD is in keeping with the clinical phenomenology of the condition, which is characterized not by a deficit state but rather by excessive mental activity directed in specific directions; repeated ruminations, mental rituals or anxiety associated with compulsive behaviours. In OCD a variety of cerebral regions have been identified showing increased activity in different studies. Rubin *et al.*[58] found no difference between patients with OCD and normal controls using the $^{133}$Xe inhalation method but when they performed the same study with $^{99m}$Tc-HMPAO they observed increased uptake in the OCD group in dorsal parietal and orbital frontal cortices bilaterally and in the left posterofrontal cortex. Another SPET-HMPAO study of 10 OCD patients demonstrated relatively increased medial frontal cortical flow but no difference in the orbital frontal region[42]. Technical differences in scanner technology may underlie the differences between these studies[33]. However, the findings of increased activity in the orbital frontal cortex have also been reported in three PET studies of regional glucose metabolism in OCD[5,6,51]. Although not all the published studies agree, there is sufficient correspondence between results to allow the formation of a neuroanatomical model of the brain systems in which dysfunction in brain regions responsible for initiating and inhibiting behaviours may lead to the development of OCD[33]. Although far from proven, the construction of this model will generate testable hypotheses, allowing the theory to develop, and it represents a good example of the unique contribution which functional imaging can make to the study of functional illness.

Unfortunately, a more common and often crippling psychiatric illness, schizophrenia, has proved resistant to investigation by functional imaging techniques. Although many abnormalities, both of cerebral perfusion and metabolism and of dopamine activity have been found in resting state studies, the absence of any consistent results have limited the conclusions that may be drawn. Currently, although great research interest remains, particularly in cognitive activation imaging of schizophrenia, there are as yet no indications for routine functional imaging as a clinical procedure in the assessment of the condition.

Imaging studies have however been of value in helping to classify the basic nature of some behavioural abnormalities. The rare but severely disabling condition of infantile autism has been variously thought of as being due to deficits in parenting skills, a purely psychological problem in the affected children or as a pervasive abnormality of brain development. Magnetic resonance imaging has provided some evidence of various structural deficits. More recently two SPET blood flow studies have demonstrated abnormalities of cerebral perfusion, particularly of temporal and frontal lobes, both at rest in adults[21] and during auditory stimulation in children[39]. These findings appear to correspond to the observed problems of speech and social interaction that characterize this condition and which have previously been localized by well-established lesion studies to temporo-frontal and frontal regions. Hence in the case of autism, SPET has provided valuable confirmatory evidence that the disease is indeed one of primary brain dysfunction, rather than an acquired disorder of social development.

## Activation studies

Activation studies in essence involve the comparison of at least two data sets describing brain activity generated in conditions that differ for the specific function in question. In normal volunteers it is possible to investigate regional and neurophysiological responses to pharmacological and behavioural challenges. In patients these techniques may be utilized to examine the effects of pathological states on specific aspects of cerebral activity.

Techniques to measure blood flow in circumscribed regions of the intact human brain were developed by Lassen and colleagues using $^{133}$Xe injected into the carotid artery[37]. Using this approach together with a gamma camera consisting of 254 externally placed scintillation detectors they were able to measure flow-determined distribution of radioactivity in the superficial cerebral cortex generated in a variety of states. From this beginning, progress in detector technology, data collection and image reconstruction and radio-tracer development has led to the current abilities for rapid three-dimensional visualization of the entire brain volume. These advances mean that SPET is now an increasingly valuable tool in the observation and analysis of cerebral response to challenges in which these responses may be distributed throughout the brain.

The SPET activation paradigms currently in vogue followed the development of $^{99m}$Tc-HMPAO. The features of this substance that lead to its utility in activation studies are in particular its rapid fixation in the brain, over a period of less than 4 min, followed by its relative stability over several hours. These properties mean that in order to measure the pattern of cerebral blood flow associated with a task, it is necessary to perform that task only during the relatively short fixation period. The subsequent stability means that, after acquiring an image following the first administration of the tracer, a subsequent image associated with a second injection of $^{99m}$Tc-HMPAO, administered during a different task, or state, may be acquired, with the results superimposed on the results of the first scan. At present the $^{99m}$Tc-HMPAO activation paradigms do not allow absolute quantification of rCBF (in ml/dl/min). Unfortunately the dose of radioactivity required to generate an adequate image generally limits the number of scans that an individual may undergo to two. However, patterns of relative change in rCBF between the two conditions may nevertheless give valuable information about task-related changes in cerebral functioning.

A number of groups around the world, using variations on this split-dose design, have performed a range of activation studies. Because the total dose to be administered is split between the two scans, these studies share the important feature that the total radiation dose to the subject is the same as it would be if they were undergoing a single clinical scan. Activation paradigms in which the two scans are performed on separate days are subject to a number of disadvantages. Firstly, such a study design generally utilizes two full doses of the radiotracer. And secondly, the prolonged interval between the two scans introduces several potentially confounding variables. These include: problems of repositioning and, particularly with reference to cognitive activations and studies of patients, changes in ambient affective state and level of arousal.

**Data analysis**

The majority of the SPET studies reviewed here have measured activity in predetermined regions of interest (ROI). In the case of resting state studies, in the absence of a measured input function with the inability to make absolute measurements of regional HMPAO uptake, comparison between subjects necessitates the calculation of a ratio of regional activity to an internal normalizing or comparative value. This approach may also be used for activation studies. In $^{99m}$Tc-HMPAO studies Goldenberg et al.[27] and Lang et al.[35] used relative count rates obtained for each of the multiple ROIs measured by dividing the tracer concentration in that region by the mean count rate of all regions taken together. In a similar approach a ratio of activity in the ROI to activity in the whole slice is calculated and it is this ratio that is used in subsequent comparisons. Matsuda et al.[43] and Battistin et al.[3] expressed activity as a ratio of activity in each ROI to the mean count rate over the cerebellum, corrected for early diffusion of tracer. None of these methods is without drawbacks. The former dilutes the size of an activation effect in any specific region whilst the latter rests on the assumption that the cerebellum is itself not activated by the test procedure. The results were then discussed either purely as size of change in flow in regions of interest between conditions[8,65], or examined for significance with $t$ tests[3,34].

In activation studies an alternative approach is to calculate activation indices for each subject, which may then be compared within and between subjects. For instance, in a study of finger movement in normal volunteers[22], an index of activation was calculated separately for six ROIs according to the formula: (task–control)/0.5(task+control).

The shape of ROIs varies. In some studies they are predetermined and regular whilst in others they are irregular and designed to enclose a specific structure. Regions may be placed in the required position either individually and manually or with the aid of a standardized computer algorithm.

Although in most studies placement of ROIs is planned before the results are obtained, in some cases authors have waited until preliminary analysis has identified the pixels of greatest change on activation, and then positioned the ROIs at this site in the images[68]. This technique precludes the possibility of a hypothesis-driven analysis and there is a danger that this method of using regions of peak change for the comparisons between conditions could bias the results towards a positive but meaningless difference between scans. In studies with several activation tasks, comparisons between stimulated conditions across individuals may be examined using analysis of variance techniques[26].

**Interpretation of results**

Investigations of individual responses of discrete brain regions are based on the assumption that higher cognitive functions are performed by distinct brain regions working independently[26]. However, many argue that the bases of higher cognitive functions arise from larger functional systems whose composition depends on the nature of the task in hand[41,62]. In this case the information of interest will be the way in which activity co-varies in functionally related brain regions. A more suitable statistical approach would then focus on correlational analyses.

Cerebral integration was first assessed in a cerebral blood flow study by Prohovnik et al.[56] using a xenon inhalation technique in resting normal volunteers. This study argued that correlation of flow rates between contralateral, homologous brain areas is an estimate of functional integration (or coupling) between the two areas. These observations were extended by Clark et al.[14] in the context of discussing the dangers implicit in taking findings of cerebral asymmetry as evidence for cerebral regional specialization. These authors, in glucose metabolism PET studies, found that coupling patterns were consistent with and dependent on stimulus states in normal subjects and that they were different in patients with schizophrenia compared with normals. They concluded that the probability of finding evidence to support a cerebral specialization model of brain function based on hemisphere asymmetry is dependent, in part, on the degree of cerebral integration when within-subject comparisons are performed. This is so because as the degree of cerebral integration increases the right/left comparisons show a smaller difference. As this correlation approaches unity any difference between right and left flow will become significant. Hence an apparent asymmetry of function may in reality be a function of strong regional integration.

In a PET study of normal volunteers Mettler et al.[47] examined correlations within 26 brain regions during resting fluorodeoxyglucose scans. Using a correlation matrix for the 26 regions of interest they identified two apparently separate functional metabolic systems. This functional interaction of brain regions is particularly relevant for more complex cognitive tasks such as language[54] where a PET study using distribution analysis provided support for a multiple, parallel route model of lexical processing. Goldenberg et al., using $^{123}$I-IMP-SPET, investigated the imagery and memorizing of words and identified the involvement of correlational structures including inferior temporal and occipital regions[26].

As pointed out by Goldenberg et al., these two statistical approaches, the search for discrete regions of changed activity, or that for patterns of correlation between regions, are not mutually exclusive techniques and the method utilized should depend on the nature of the function being investigated. For more complex tasks correlational analysis is more likely to contribute important information about the neural basis of performance whilst for studies primarily investigating specific aspects of cerebral blood flow[15,43] the search for significant change in specific regions may be more relevant.

With respect to the nature of models of cerebral processing, it has been pointed out[36] that, because of the enormous complexity of the brain, descriptions of its function have tended to be formulated in terms of the most sophisticated technology of the day; from ideas of aqueduct-like flows of bodily humours in ancient Greece and Rome, through Sherrington's analogy of a telephone switchboard, to modern concepts based on computer models of artificial intelligence. Recent ideas have progressed from ideas of serial processing of information along a hierarchy of dedicated centres. Now theories of parallel-distributed processing (PDP) based in interconnected neural networks[45,46,59] are generating increasing interest and have been proposed as a theoretical template for the interpretation of a number of activation studies[13,54,55,67].

SPECT activation paradigms have been used explicitly to explore models of cerebral processing.

Demonet *et al.*[17], in a carefully designed study, looked for difference in patterns of cerebral blood flow (CBF) associated with changes in the semantic coherence of sentences. In particular they wished to distinguish patterns associated with parallel processing in coherent sentences from serial processing in non-coherent circumstances. In fact they failed to demonstrate any significant changes in CBF across conditions.

The authors did however detect condition-specific differences in the pattern of correlations across regions. The primary assumption for such an analysis is that neural units that function together will have changes in activity that are correlated[30]. Given the evidence that multiple brain regions interact in complex behaviours, functional neuroimaging provides a unique means of dissecting out task-specific cerebral systems. In this context, the nature of the theoretical models employed to interpret the results of imaging studies assume great importance.

### Activation studies in normal volunteers

Early projects focused on simple motor activation tasks. The purpose of these was to validate the technique by comparing the results with the known neurophysiology of motor control. This has been demonstrated both for a ratio of first to second dose of 1:1[23] and for a ratio of 1:3[52]. Other studies have also investigated the use of rest:task dose ratios of 1:2[29], or 1:3[69].

The normal cerebral representation of other basic neurophysiological processes have been investigated using $^{99m}$Tc-HMPAO in a double-dose, separate-day imaging paradigm. Visual activation using stroboscopic photic stimulation demonstrated the expected increase in radiopharmaceutical distribution to the visual cortex[68]. Le Scao *et al.*[38] explored the effects of tonal stimulation on the auditory pathways. They observed that stimulation resulted in increases of temporal perfusion of 17–19 per cent.

Rates of rCBF associated with a particular task are determined by local neuronal activity[57] which itself is determined by the manner in which the brain performs the task. In these circumstances a result that at one level is an indication of the physical location of a function, at another is indicative of the nature of the work performed by the brain in the performance of the task. This reasoning has led to the use of activation paradigms which seek to explore the cerebral basis of more sophisticated, higher cognitive functions.

The use of a cognitively complex task, the Stroop attentional conflict paradigm, has demonstrated activation of a number of mainly left-sided brain areas[11,53]. The most robust response however was in the anterior cingulate cortex. Clear activations were not observed in corresponding right-sided regions. This may be because the task involved the visual presentation of words, likely to activate left-hemisphere structures in the right-handed subjects of this study. Nevertheless, it is possible to combine the results of these two studies to suggest that a human attentional system may involve the anterior cingulate cortex and right-sided pre-frontal and superior parietal cortices.

In a series of studies, Goldenberg and colleagues investigated the cerebral basis of visual imagery[25 –28]. In particular they wished to address the question of whether the introspective experience of having mental visual images corresponded to a distinct mode of cognitive processing. A number of experimental paradigms were employed. Subjects were investigated during rest and whilst memorizing abstract, concrete or meaningless words with and without the instruction to use visual memory as an *aide-mémoire*. In later studies the imaging of faces, colours and maps were compared and the role of cognitive tasks which either did or did not require visual imagery were investigated. When interpreting their studies a number of technical and task-related difficulties must be borne in mind. As the authors point out, it is not possible to completely control or suppress acts of visual imagery. Hence during both resting and auditory imaging states, the subjects subsequently reported the occurrence of spontaneous visual images. Thus even if sensory imaging were based in modality-specific structures it would not be possible to demonstrate a double-dissociation between auditory and visual imagery. In addition the paradigms utilized may involve other functions such as linguistic analysis, memory and emotional response to the stimuli. With respect to analysis of the SPECT images, the limited anatomical information derived from the blood-flow images renders it difficult to localize the anatomical site of findings of interest. Indeed this is true for functional neuroimaging studies in general. Nevertheless, combining the results from these studies allowed the authors to conclude that whilst there is no 'imagery centre', there is support for the hypothesis that the cerebral correlates of visual imagery, involving inferior temporal and occipital regions, are different from that of non-imaginal thinking.

**Activation studies in patients**

There have been fewer activation studies in patients with neuropsychiatric states than there have been in normals and this paradigm has not yet earned a role in routine clinical management. However there have been several investigations of regional brain activity in schizophrenia. The aim of these studies was to investigate the cerebral basis of schizophrenic symptoms. A SPET study of schizophrenic patients performing a verbal fluency task that is thought to involve frontal lobe structures, demonstrated that compared to a control group, the schizophrenic sample had decreased HMPAO uptake in left frontal cortical and left posterior cortical regions[40]. Unfortunately this study did not include a control condition so it is not possible to interpret the results as validating the failure of frontal lobe activation demonstrated by Weinberger & Berman using [133]Xe inhalation and a different frontal lobe task[66]. However, the observation by Lewis et al.[40] that there was a correlation between the severity of the negative symptoms experienced by their schizophrenic patients and left medial frontal blood flow agrees with several other studies suggesting that dysfunction of this brain region is associated with the avolitional elements of schizophrenia.

Pharmacological activation studies may be used to learn about the cerebral actions of the administered drug. Alternatively the known cerebral effects of a substance that requires or activates specific brain regions or functions may allow examination of these particular systems. Thus an investigation into cholinergic involvement in the memory deficits of Alzheimer's dementia[3] utilized the cholinomimetic properties of L-acetylcarnitine to observe the effects of increasing cholinergic activity on regional, particularly parietal, cerebral blood flow in patients with this condition.

Two studies have investigated the effect of the anticholinesterase, physostigmine, on patterns of regional cerebral blood flow. Unfortunately this drug has not proved to be effective in the treatment of Alzheimer's dementia although both studies reported that its administration was associated with regional increases in tracer uptake. In a study without a control group it appeared that physostigmine increased uptake in frontoparietal regions as measured by cortical:white matter activity ratios in five dementing patients[32]. However, in two further patients injection of saline produced a similar result. Using the calculation of an asymmetry index it also appeared that physostigmine produced an increase in tracer uptake in the left hemisphere relative to the right. Although there is some evidence of asymmetry of markers of pathology in Alzheimer's disease, it is not currently possible to derive clinical utility from these results. Nevertheless, the effect of physostigmine in increasing [99m]Tc-HMPAO uptake in brain regions involved in this condition was also demonstrated in an experiment comparing the effects of the drug in a sample with Alzheimer's disease and in normal controls[20]. In this study it was observed that the pharmacological challenge was associated with focal increases in tracer uptake in posterior parieto-temporal regions in the patients but not in the controls.

Pharmacological techniques provide a new means for investigating cerebrovascular disease. A number of studies have examined the results of challenging the cerebral vasculature with substances that have vasodilating effects. Dahl *et al.*[15] examined the response to nitroglycerine in dilating cerebral vasculature in part as an investigation into the therapeutic actions of this drug. Other substances having similar effects have also been utilized in activation paradigms. The inhalation of 7 per cent carbon dioxide may produce side-effects such as nausea, tachycardia and increased blood pressure[16]. Acetazolamide on the other hand is a powerful but harmless vasodilator that exerts its effects within 10 min following intravenous injection[12,16], increasing regional cerebral blood flow in normal tissue by approximately 35 per cent[2]. It has been used to study cerebral blood flow reactivity in patients with transient ischaemic attacks (TIAs)[12], significantly increasing the sensitivity of SPET for detecting regions of pathological blood flow. The technique has also enabled the demonstration of hypoperfusion and impaired vasoreactivity in occipital and cerebellar regions in a patient with vertebrobasilar insufficiency[16].

## Conclusions

The observation in intact humans of local changes in cerebral blood flow during the performance of specific behaviours or tasks gives an indication of ongoing regional brain activity associated with these states. Such information is not currently obtainable by other modes of investigation.

In attempting to assess the meaning of such results, a number of points must be considered. These include the proposition that complex human behaviours reside not at a single locus but rather that they emerge from the inter-related activity of a number of cerebral structures. In addition, any particular structure may be involved in more than one behaviour and may· at different times act in concert with a variable number of the other structures to which it is connected. These intricate networks are obviously only currently amenable to a coarse level of analysis.

In the future, developments in new techniques to observe task-related changes in regional cerebral blood flow will improve temporal and spatial resolution. The ability to co-register data from functional neuroimaging and magnetic resonance imaging will improve the anatomical localization available to the former technique. Refinement of theoretical models of brain functioning are also critical if the most is to be made of these technical innovations.

The choice of simple and well-controlled activation paradigms have yielded results in sensory, motor and cognitive paradigms that are both consistent with existing knowledge and appropriate to interpretation by recent models of cerebral information processing. The analysis of emotional and other abstract mental properties such as depression, hallucinations and thought disorder is more difficult. This may be because these processes have a more diffuse cerebral representation or it may be that in common with other modes of psychiatric research, the difficulty in defining a meaningfully homogenous study population limits successful research. With respect to neuropsychiatry, the goals of identifying cerebral correlates of psychopathology and the nature of their association with demonstrable brain disease remain to be achieved. However, the success of activation studies in the investigation of normal psychological and physiological processes, and the ability of resting state examinations of psychiatric disease, albeit with discrepancies between studies, to display regional functional disturbances associated with particular psychopathological states, suggest that the activation approach in neuropsychiatry may bear more fruit in the future.

## Acknowledgements

I am grateful for financial support from the Raymond Way Memorial Fund.

# References

1.  Adams, R.D. & Victor, M. (1985): *Principles of neurology*. New York: McGraw Hill.

2.  Batjer, H.H., Devous, M.D., Meyer, M.J., Purdy, P.D. & Samson, D.S. (1988): Cerebrovascular haemodynamics in arteriovenous malformation complicated by normal perfusion pressure breakthrough. *Neurosurgery* **22**, 503–509.

3.  Battisstin, L., Pizzolato, G., Dam, M., Da Col, C., Perlotto, N., Saitta, B., Borsato, N., Calvani, M. & Ferlin, G. (1989): Single-photon emission computed tomography studies with $^{99m}$Tc-hexamethylpropyleneamine oxime in dementia: effects of acute administration of L-acetylcarnitine. *Eur. Neurol.* **29**, 261–265.

4.  Baxter, L.R. (1990): Brain imaging as a tool in establishing a theory of brain pathology in obsessive compulsive disorder. *J. Clin. Psychiatry* **51(S)**, 22–25.

5.  Baxter, L.R., Phelps, M.E., Mazziota, J.C., Guze, G.H., Schwartz, J.M., Gerner, R.H. & Selin, C.E. (1987): Local cerebral glucose metabolic rates in obsessive-compulsive disorder. *Arch. Gen. Psychiatry* **44**, 211–218.

6.  Baxter, L.R., Schwartz, J.M., Mazziotta, J.C., Phelps, M.E., Pahl, J.J., Guze, B.H. & Fairbanks, L. (1988): Cerebral glucose metabolic rates in non-depressed patients with obsessive-compulsive disorder. *Am. J. Psychiatry* **145**, 1560–1563.

7.  Bench, C.J., Friston, K.J., Brown, R.G., Scott, L.C., Frackowiak, R.S.J. & Dolan, R.J. (1992): The anatomy of melancholia – focal abnormalities of cerebral blood flow in major depression and the cognitive impairment of depression. *Psychol. Med.* **22**, 607–615.

8.  Biersack, H.J., Linke, D., Brassel, F., Reichman, K., Kurhten, M., Durwen, H.F., Reuter, B.M., Wappenschmidt, J. & Stefan, H. (1987): Tc-99m-HMPAO brain SPECT in epileptic patients before and during unilateral hemispheric anesthesia (Wada test), Report of three cases. *J. Nucl. Med.* **28**, 1763–1767.

9.  Brown, R.G. & Marsden, C.D. (1984): How common is dementia in Parkinson's disease? *Lancet* **ii**, 1262–1265.

10. Burns, A., Philpot, M.P., Costa, D.C. *et al.* (1989): The investigation of Alzheimer's disease with single photon emission tomography. *J. Neurol. Neurosurg. Psychiatry* **52**, 248–253.

11. Camargo, E.E., Rivera-Luna, H., Sostre, S., Hoehn-Saric, R., Pearlson, G.D., McLeod, D.R., Szabo, Z., Madary, J., Harris, G. & Wagner, H.N. Jr. (1991): Cerebral activation during the Stroop test identified by brain SPECT imaging. *Eur. J. Nucl. Med.* **18**, 595 (abstr.)

12. Chollet, F., Celsis, P., Clanet, M., Guiraud-Chaumeil, B. & Marc-Vergnes, J.-P. (1989): SPECT study of cerebral blood flow reactivity after acetazolamide in patients with transient ischaemic attacks. *Stroke* **20**, 458–464.

13. Chollet, F., DiPiero, V., Wise, R.J.S., Brooks, D.J., Dolan, R.J. & Frackowiak, R.S.J. (1991): The functional anatomy of motor recovery after stroke in humans: a study with positron emission tomography. *Ann. Neurol.* **29**, 63–71.

14. Clark, C.M., Kessler, R. & Margolin, R. (1985): The statistical interaction of cerebral specialization and integration in the interpretation of dynamic brain images. *Brain Cognit.* **4**, 7–12.

15. Dahl, A., Russel, D., Nyberg-Hansen, R., & Rootwelt, K. (1989): Effect of nitroglycerin on cerebral circulation measured by transcranial Doppler and SPECT. *Stroke* **20**, 1733–1736.

16. Delecluse, F., Voordecker, P. & Raftopoulos, C. (1989): Vertebrobasilar insufficiency revealed by xenon-133 inhalation SPECT. *Stroke* **20**, 952–956.

17. Demonet, J.-F., Celsis, P., Nespoulous, J.-L., Viallard, G., Marc-Vergnes, J.-P., & Rascol, A. (1992): Cerebral blood flow correlates of word monitoring in sentences: influences of semantic incoherence. A SPECT study in normals. *Neuropsychologia* **30**, 1–11.

18. Deutsch, G. (1992): The nonspecificity of frontal dysfunction in disease and altered states: cortical blood flow evidence. *Neuropsychiat. Neuropsychol. Behav. Neurol.* **5**, 301–307.

19. Fox, P.T. (1989): Functional brain mapping with positron emission tomography. *Semin. Neurol.* **9**, 323–329.

20. Geaney, D.P., Soper, N., Shepstone, B.J. & Cowen, P.J. (1990): Effect of central cholinergic stimulation on regional cerebral blood flow in Alzheimer disease. *Lancet* **335**, 1484–1487.

21.  George, M.S., Costa, D.C., Kouris, K. Ring, H.A. & Ell, P.J. (1992): Cerebral blood flow abnormalities in adults with infantile autism. *J. Nerv. Ment. Dis.* **180**, 413–417 (abstr.)

22.  George, M.S., Ring, H.A., Costa, D.C., Ell, P.J., Kouris, K. & Jarritt, P.H. (1991): *Neuroactivation and neuroimaging with SPET*. London: Springer Verlag.

23.  George, M.S., Ring, H.A., Costa, D.C., Kouris, K. & Ell, P.J. (1992): Demonstration of human motor cortex activation using SPECT. *J. Neural Trans.* **87**, 231–236.

24.  Goldenberg, G., Podreka, I., Pfaffelmeyer, N., Wessely, P. & Deecke, L. (1991): Thalamic ischaemia in transient global amnesia: a SPECT study. *Neurology* **41**, 1748–1752.

25.  Goldenberg, G., Podreka, I., Steiner, M., Franzen, P. & Deecke, L. (1991): Contributions of occipital and temporal brain regions to visual and acoustic imagery – a SPECT study. *Neuropsychologia* **29**, 695–702.

26.  Goldenberg, G., Podreka, I., Steiner, M. & Willmes, K. (1987): Patterns of regional cerebral blood flow related to memorizing of high and low imagery words – an emission computer tomography study. *Neuropsychologia* **25**, 473–485.

27.  Goldenberg, G., Podreka, I., Steiner, M., Willmes, K., Seuss, E. & Deecke, L. (1989): Regional cerebral blood flow patterns in visual imagery. *Neuropsychologia* **27**, 641–664.

28.  Goldenberg, G., Podreka, I., Uhl, F., Steiner, M., Willmes, K. & Deecke, L. (1989): Cerebral correlates of imagining colours, faces and a map. I. SPECT of regional cerebral blood flow. *Neuropsychologia* **27**, 1315–1328.

29.  Holm, S., Madsen, P.L., Rubin, P., Sperling, B., Friberg, L. & Lassen, N.A. (1991): $^{99m}$Tc-HMPAO activation studies: validation of the split-dose, image subtraction approach. *J. Cereb. Blood Flow Metab.* **11**, Suppl.2, S766 (abstr.)

30.  Horwitz, B. (1991): Functional interactions in the brain: use of correlations between regional metabolic rates. *J. Cereb. Blood Flow Metab.* **11**, A114–A120.

31.  Hunter, R., McLuskie, R., Wyper, D., Patterson, J., Christie, J.E., Brooks, D.N., McCullough, J., Fink, G. & Goodwin, G.M. (1989): The pattern of function-related regional cerebral blood flow investigated by single photon emission tomography with $^{99m}$Tc-HMPAO in patients with presenile Alzheimer's disease and Korsakoff's psychosis. *Psychol. Med.* **19**, 847–855.

32.  Hunter, R., Wyper, D.J., Patterson, J., Hansen, M.T. & Goodwin, G.M. (1991): Cerebral pharmacodynamics of physostigmine in Alzheimer's disease investigated using single-photon computerised tomography. *Br. J. Psychiatry* **158**, 357.

33.  Insel, T.R. (1992): Toward a neuroanatomy of obsessive-compulsive disorder. *Arch. Gen. Psychiatry* **49**, 739–744

34.  Lang, W., Lang, M., Podreka, I., Steiner, M., Uhl, F., Suess, E., Muller, Ch. & Deecke, L. (1988): DC-potential shifts and regional cerebral blood flow reveal frontal cortex involvement in human visuomotor learning. *Exp. Brain Res.* **71**, 353–364.

35.  Lang, W., Podreka, I., Suess, E., Muller, C., Zeitlhofer, J. & Deecke, L. (1988): Single photon emission computerized tomography during and between seizures. *J. Neurol.* **235**, 277–284.

36.  Lashley, K.S. (1937): Functional determinants of cerebral localization. *Arch. Neurol. Psychiatry* **38**, 371–387.

37.  Lassen, N.A., Ingvar, D.H. & Skinhoj, E. (1978): Brain function and blood flow. *Sci. Am.* **239**, 50–59.

38.  Le Scao, Y., Baulieu, J.L., Robier, A., Pourcelot, L. & Beutter, P. (1991): Increment of brain temporal perfusion during auditory stimulation. *Eur. J. Nucl. Med.* **18**, 981–983.

39.  Lelord, G., Garreau, B., Syrota, A., Bruneau, N., Pourcelot, L. & Zilbovicius, M. (1991): SPECT rCBF, Doppler transcranial ultrasonography and evoked potential studies in pervasive developmental disorders. *Biol. Psychiatry* **29**, 292s.

40.  Lewis, S.H., Ford, R.A., Syed, G.M., Reveley, A.M. & Toone, B.K. (1992): A controlled study of $^{99m}$Tc-HMPAO single-photon emission imaging in chronic schizophrenia. *Psychol. Med.* **22**, 27–35.

41.  Luria, A.R. (1980): *Higher cortical functions in man*. New York: Basic Books.

42.  Machlin, S.R., Harris, G.J., Pearlson, G.D., Hoehn-Saric, R., Jeffery, P. & Camargo, E.E. (1991): Elevated medial-frontal cerebral blood flow in obsessive-compulsive patients: a SPECT study. *Am. J. Psychiatry* **148**, 1240–1242.

43.  Matsuda, H., Higashi, S., Asli, I.N., Eftekhari, M., Esmaili, J., Seki, H., Tsuji, S., Oba, H., Imai, K., Terada, H., Sumiya, H. & Hisada, K. (1988): Evaluation of cerebral collateral circulation by Tc-99m-HMPAO brain SPECT during Matas test: report of three cases. *J. Nucl. Med.* **29**, 1724–1729.

44.  Mayberg, H.S., Starkstein, S.E., Sadzot, B., Preziosi, T.J., Andrezejewski, P.L., Dannals, R.F., Wagner, H.N. & Robinson, R.G. (1990): Selective hypometabolism in the inferior frontal lobe in depressed patients with Parkinson's disease. *Ann. Neurol.* **28**, 57–64.

45.  McClelland, J.L., Rumelhart, D.E. & The PDP Research Group (1986): *Parallel distributed processing.* Volume 2. Cambridge, Massachusetts: MIT Press.

46.  Mesulam, M.-M. (1990): Large-scale neurocognitive networks and distributed processing for attention, language and memory. *Ann. Neurol.* **28**, 597–613.

47.  Mettler, E.J., Riege, W.H., Kuhl, D.E. & Phelps, M.E. (1984): Cerebral metabolic relationships for selected brain regions in healthy adults. *J. Cereb. Blood Flow Metab.* **4**, 1–7.

48.  Miller, B.L., Cummings, J.L., Villanueva-Meyer, J., Boone, K., Mehringer, C.M., Lesser, I.M. & Mena, I. (1991): Frontal lobe degeneration: clinical, neuropsychological, and SPECT characteristics. *Neurology* **41**, 1374–1382.

49.  Neary, D., Snowden, J.S., Northen, B. & Goulding, P. (1988): Dementia of frontal lobe type. *J. Neurol. Neurosurg. Psychiatry* **51**, 353–361.

50.  Neary, D., Snowden, J.S., Shields, R.A., Burjan, A.W.I., Northen, B., Macdermott, N., Prescot, M.C. & Testa, H.J. (1987): Single photon emission tomography using [99m]Tc-HMPAO in the investigation of dementia. *J. Neurol. Neurosurg. Psychiatry* **50**, 1101–1109.

51.  Nordahl, T.E., Benkelfat, C., Semple, W.E. *et al.* (1989): Cerebral glucose metabolic rates in obsessive-compulsive disorder. *Neuropsychopharmacology* **2**, 23–28 (abstr.)

52.  Pantano, P., Lenzi, G.L., Di Piero, V., Ricci, M. & Fieschi, C. (1991): CBF-SPECT activation study by [99m]Tc-HM-PAO split-dose method. *J. Cereb. Blood Flow Metab.* **11**, Suppl. 2, S767 (abstr.)

53.  Pardo, J.V, Pardo, P.J., Janer, K.W. & Raichle, M.E. (1990): The anterior cingulate cortex mediates processing selection in the Stroop attentional conflict paradigm. *Proc. Natl. Acad. Sci. USA* **87**, 256–259.

54.  Petersen, S.E., Fox, P.T., Posner, M.I., Mintum, M. & Raichle, M.E. (1988): Positron emission tomographic studies of the cortical anatomy of single-word processing. *Nature* **331**, 585–589.

55.  Posner, M.I., Petersen, S.E., Fox, P.T. & Raichle, M.E. (1988): Localization of cognitive operations in the human brain. *Science* **240**, 1627–1631.

56.  Prohovnik, I., Hakansson, K. & Risberg, J. (1980): Observations on the functional significance of regional cerebral blood flow in 'resting' normal subjects. *Neuropsychologia* **18**, 203–217.

57.  Raichle, M.E. (1990): Developing a functional anatomy of the human visual system with positron emission tomography. In: *Vision and the brain*, edited by B. Cohen, , pp. 257–270. New York: Raven Press.

58.  Rubin, R.T., Villanueva-Meyer, J., Ananth, J., Trajmar, P.G. & Mena, I. (1992): Regional xenon-133 cerebral blood flow and cerebral technetium-99m HMPAO uptake in unmedicated patients with obsessive compulsive disorder and matched normal control subjects. *Arch. Gen Psychiatry* **49**, 695–702.

59.  Rumelhart, D.E., McClelland, J.L. & The PDP Research Group (1986): *Parallel distributed processing.* Volume 1. Cambridge, Massachusetts: MIT Press.

60.  Spampinato, U., Habert, M.O., Mas, J.L., Bourdel, M.C., Ziegler, M., de Recondo, J., Askienazy, S. & Rondot, P. (1991): [99m]Tc-HMPAO SPECT and cognitive impairment in Parkinson's disease: a comparison with dementia of the Alzheimer type. *J. Neurol. Neurosurg. Psychiatry* **54**, 787–792.

61.  Stilhard, G., Landis, T., Schiess, R., Regard, M. & Sialer, G. (1990): Bitemporal hypoperfusion in transient global amnesia: [99m]Tc-HMPAO SPECT and neuropsychological findings during and after an attack. *J. Neurol. Neurosurg. Psychiatry* **53**, 339–342.

62.  Stuss, D.T. & Benson, D.F. (1986): *The frontal lobes.* New York: Raven Press.

63.  Swedo, S.E., Schapiro, M.B., Grady, C.L., Cheslow, D.L., Leonard, H.L., Kumar, A., Friedland, R., Rapoport, S.I. & Rapoport, J.L. (1989): Cerebral glucose metabolism in childhood-onset obsessive compulsive disorder. *Arch. Gen. Psych.* **46**, 518–523.

64.  Taylor, A., Saint-Cyr, J.A. & Lang, A.E. (1985): Dementia prevalence in Parkinson's disease. *Lancet* **i**, 1037.

65.    Walker-Batson, D., Wendt, J.S., Devous, M.D., Barton, M.M. & Bonte, F.J. (1988): A long-term followup case study of crossed aphasia assessed by single-photon emission tomography (SPECT), language, and neuropsychological testing. *Brain Lang.* **33**, 311–322.

66.    Weinberger, D.R., Berman, K.F. & Zec, R.F. (1986): Physiologic dysfunction of dorsolateral prefrontal cortex in schizophrenia. *Arch. Gen. Psych.* **43**, 114–124.

67.    Wise, R., Chollet, F., Hadar, U., Friston, K., Hoffner, E. & Frackowiak, R.S.J. (1991): Distribution of cortical neural networks involved in word comprehension and word retrieval. *Brain* **114**, 1803–1817.

68.    Woods, S.W., Hegeman, I.M., Zubal, I.G., Krystal, J.H., Koster, K., Smith, E.O., Heninger, G.R. & Hoffer, P.B. (1991): Visual stimulation increases Tc-99m-HMPAO distribution in human visual cortex. *J. Nucl. Med.* **32**, 210–215.

69.    Wyper, D.J., Hunter, R., Patterson, J., Goodwin, G. & McCulloch, J. (1991): A split-dose technique for measuring changes in cerebral blood flow patterns. *J. Cereb. Blood Flow Metab.* **11**, Suppl. 2, S449 (abstr.)

*New Trends in Nuclear Neurology and Psychiatry*, edited by D.C. Costa, G.F. Morgan and N. A. Lassen
© 1993 John Libbey & Company Ltd., pp. 133–149

# Chapter 9

# Non-invasive brain imaging techniques (SPET, PET and MRI): relative merits and synergistic use

Giovanni Lucignani, Giovanna Rizzo, [1]Fabio Triulzi,
Maria Carla Gilardi, Cristina Messa, Rosa Maria Moresco,
Giovanni Paganelli, [1]Giuseppe Scotti and Ferruccio Fazio

*INB-CNR, Department of Nuclear Medicine and [1]Department of Neuroradiology, University of Milan,
Scientific Institute H. San Raffaele, Milan, Italy*

## Introduction

**M**ethods of structural and functional imaging, including X-ray computed tomography (X-ray CT), magnetic resonance (MR), and emission tomography (ET) allow the assessment of some morphological, biochemical, and physiological characteristics of the central nervous system. These methods have a considerable impact in the diagnostic work-up, staging, therapeutic planning, interventional therapy, and follow-up of patients with neurological diseases. Several different imaging methods can currently be used in a specific and orderly chronological sequence for diagnostic purposes. The same methods are also employed systematically to examine challenging issues in neurochemistry, neuropharmacology and neurophysiology.

The information acquired with the various imaging modalities is often complementary; therefore, it is a current procedure to exploit the potentials of two or more imaging modalities in order to obtain more accurate information and new insight on the status and function of an organ. The collation of the information obtained with different modalities is usually the clinician's task. However, due to the developments in the area of biomedical imaging technology (BIT), a new strategy aimed at the synergistic use of the different BITs is evolving. This is, for example, the case of the integration of MR imaging, for the definition of anatomical landmarks around and within an organ, with ET by which physiological or biochemical processes are examined. In particular, integration and registration of BITs is crucial for the analysis of functional images with a poorly defined anatomical pattern, such as those of receptor and immunoscintigraphic studies, and for the evaluation of anatomo-functional variables, i.e. tissue heterogeneity and atrophy, that may hamper the correct measurement of biochemical and physiological processes when they are overlooked.

Although the choice of specific methods to be used in the investigation of patients with neurological diseases must remain, in principle, selective and sequential, new information can be obtained without any further patient involvement at the little additional cost necessary for the fusion of individual images, by correlating and integrating information obtained with two or more imaging devices and methods. Inasmuch as the synergistic strategy allows us to gain a more complete understanding of any given physiological, pharmacological or pathological process it could represent the basis for the modification of current diagnostic procedures. The synergistic use of the available BITs is also crucial for an effective diagnostic process and economic use of the available technology; therefore, this is an issue that can have a relevant economical and social impact and that should be considered by the medical equipment manufacturers in targeting and optimizing their products.

## Instrumentation and image integration

### Instrumentation

In the evaluation of the potentials of each imaging modality, whether for scientific research or in the process of defining an optimal diagnostic protocol, one must consider some essential physical features of the instruments available including:

(1) spatial resolution;

(2) contrast resolution;

(3) temporal resolution;

(4) short-term repeatability of the examination.

At the present time the highest spatial resolution is provided by X-ray CT and MRI. This feature is of obvious importance in the examination of any organ, but in the examination of brain morphology and function it becomes essential for differentiating contiguous yet distinct anatomo-functional structures. Furthermore, poor spatial resolution results in loss of quantitative accuracy due to partial volume effect in ET, and the assessment of tracer kinetics in the region of interest containing mixtures of different tissues may result in gross errors if functional heterogeneity is overlooked[35,67]. Several SPET dedicated systems have been developed, characterized by a large extension of the detection surface around the patient, to improve both spatial resolution and detection efficiency. With three head systems or annular rings, spatial resolution of 7–8 mm can be obtained, while sensitivity increases by a factor of three or more with respect to single head rotating gamma-cameras[9,26,41]. Further information can be obtained from Chapter 4. Current PET scanners are characterized by a spatial resolution of 4–5 mm and by multi-slice capability, covering an axial field of view of up to 15 cm or more. Despite these technological improvements, sensitivity is poor (less than 1 per cent) and this represents a limiting factor in several studies (e.g. paediatrics, pharmacokinetics, activation studies). An improvement of sensitivity can be obtained by increasing the axial acceptance angle and adopting a three-dimensional acquisition strategy. A technique has been developed for conventional scanners, based on the removal of the inter-plane septa, originally introduced to reduce scatter and random events, that allows collection of all possible coincident events by detector elements[4,70,77]. A full three-dimensional sampling of the radioactivity distribution is thus obtained and an increase in sensitivity by a factor of 5 is achieved.

The contrast resolution of MRI is superior to that of X-ray CT and can be further enhanced, both in MRI and X-ray CT by use of contrast agents and in MRI by use of different pulse sequences[29]. In nuclear medicine an improvement to signal-to-noise ratio can be achieved by optimizing the instrumentation performance, the choice of the tracer and the time of acquisition, by allowing enough time for the uptake of the tracer in the target organ and for its systemic clearance, i.e. by taking advantage of the kinetics and biodistribution of the tracers used.

The temporal resolution may be irrelevant when studying non-dynamic processes, such as the brain morphology, when the subject examined is collaborative, whereas it becomes crucial in the examination of dynamic processes such as during brain activation studies and when the subjects examined cannot remain motionless. Continuous rotation is now possible with state of the art X-ray CT scanners by the use of slip ring technology, and image acquisitions can be accomplished in times on the order of 1 s. Helicoidal (spiral) rotation is a feature of most current generation tomographs. The time necessary for ET studies is dependent upon the dose of tracer administered and it is shorter for acquisitions carried out with dedicated gamma-cameras than with general purpose instruments.

The temporal resolution of MRI is achieved both with hardware and software development and time required for scanning ranges from the few minutes of conventional spin-echo sequences, to the 30–100 msec of echoplanar imaging (EPI) techniques[72]. The availability of very intense gradients up to 30 mT/m makes possible very fast acquisition sequences, e.g. those necessary for EPI, adequate for the *in vivo* assessment of physiological processes. EPI and other fast sequences have changed the perspective of MRI and 'MRI functional imaging' is an emerging area of research.

While X-ray CT and nuclear medicine studies are limited by the radiation exposure, and in nuclear medicine also by the time necessary for decay of the tracers employed, fundamental studies on the safety of MRI are still very limited, however, the results of the studies available so far do not indicate any limitation in the repeatability of the MRI examination[68].

### Multimodality image integration and registration

The integration of images obtained with different modalities requires the achievement of three main goals:

(a) efficient and fast data transfer by networks that link different acquisition devices to central processing workstations;

(b) standardization of procedures for management of images obtained with different devices;

(c) implementation of techniques for point by point registration of morphological and functional images.

Data transfer from acquisition devices to workstations dedicated to analysis, for the purpose of integrating images obtained with different modalities, requires the handling of large volumes of data. Thus, digital data sets, on the order of Mbytes for each tomographic study, are acquired and reconstructed with computer systems that must be connected by a local network in order to ensure a fast data transfer; the use of a local network allows the independence of each system, and the data transfer can occur without interference in the acquisition process. An essential step is the decodification and conversion to a standard format (i.e. matrix size, pixel depth and file header architecture) of all digital images acquired with different modalities and instruments. Following the guidelines of the American College of Radiology (ACR) and of the National Electrical Manufacturers' Association (NEMA), several manufacturers of imaging devices have adopted standards for interfacing hardware as well as a number of software commands and data formats.

Several strategies have been implemented to achieve the registration of images obtained with different imaging modalities. The organ under examination is represented, in each of the different tomographic scanners, as a volume in a spatial co-ordinate system specific for that acquisition system. To achieve the registration of images obtained with different tomographic devices it is necessary to establish a point by point correspondence of the same anatomical-functional structures, thus, the different image volumes must be remapped in a unique reference space.

Registration techniques are used for the estimation of transformation parameters among various studies. The most common strategy for image registration is based on the use of external markers for reference to determine the image registration parameters[32,50]. The markers, made of selected radioactive or contrast agents, can be either positioned directly on the patient's skin or fixed to a device used for patient positioning[7]. A minimization algorithm is then used to estimate the best geometric transformation to overlap the markers' position in the different image volumes[2]. This strategy can be adopted in a wide range of clinical studies, but it is limited by the need of a predefined acquisition protocol, and the accuracy of the method is strictly related to the precision of the marker repositioning. A similar method, based on internal anatomical markers, has been proposed by Evans *et al.*[20] to correlate PET and MRI cerebral images; with this method 16 homologous cortical and subcortical landmarks are identified in the images to be correlated. The use of such internal landmarks allows a retrospective registration, but it can be applied only to those imaging modalities in which several homologous anatomical structures can consistently be identified in the studies to be correlated. Another strategy that allows a retrospective registration of MRI, X-ray CT and PET cerebral images has been developed by Pelizzari *et al.*[60]; the method, based on the use of an algorithm for non-linear least squares fitting, is aimed at matching the anatomical surfaces of the volumes to be correlated. However, with this method the uniqueness of the solution is not ensured due to the intrinsic limitation of non-linear minimization algorithms. All the above techniques are highly interactive and are inevitably affected by the objectivity and the experience of the user. Fully automated registration techniques that are based on the pixel-by-pixel analysis of the image characteristics have been proposed to overcome this limitation, at least for registration of studies performed with the same modality[82]. These techniques are based on the hypothesis that two studies performed with the same modality produce images with the same morphological characteristics. These techniques seem to be very powerful for the registration of studies acquired with the same acquisition modality (i.e. in PET follow-up, test-retest and activation studies), their implementation for a multimodality application is in the process of validation. All registration strategies present advantages and limitations: the choice of a particular method is strictly related to the specific clinical integration protocol. These methods are, however, prototypes that do not have a widespread clinical application as yet, since their use requires a careful planning of the various studies according to protocols that may be impractical in clinical routine situations.

## Biochemical and pharmacological imaging

### Biochemical imaging

ET and MR spectroscopy (MRS) allow the *in vivo* assessment of biochemical variables directly in the organ under examination. By using these techniques it is possible to overcome the limitations due to the indirect assessment of metabolic processes by measurements of the concentrations of metabolites and drugs in the body fluids. ET and MRS provide different yet complementary information. By using ET it is possible to quantify the concentration of radioactively labelled substances present in the organ examined in nanomolar amounts. However, ET allows only the measurement of the total concentration of radioactive molecules, and it does not distinguish among the various chemical species that may be labelled, i.e. neither the precursor nor any of the possible labelled products. Therefore strategies must be developed that ensure that the radioactivity measured at the time of the study is contained exclusively in the precursor and/or in the products specific to the chemical reaction to be assayed. The labelled precursor must be so selected that its chemical transformations are limited only to the pathway under study within the organ examined. An example of the application of this principle is provided by the deoxyglucose method, based on the measurement of the rate of formation of one product substance only, i.e. deoxyglucose-6-phosphate, and on the almost complete clearance of the precursor, i.e. free deoxyglucose, from the organ examined at the time of measurement by ET[36,69]. Additional problems are encountered with SPET, as compared to PET, due to the use of tracers labelled with radioactive isotopes of atoms that are not naturally occurring in the body. In contrast with ET, MRS can distinguish the different metabolites formed following the administration of a molecule, although the accurate quantitation of metabolite concentration is not feasible directly with conventional pulse sequences and the exact localization of the signal source may be difficult[76]. Moreover, the relatively low sensitivity of MRS is the crucial limiting factor and non-physiological amounts of exogenous tracer substance must be used, in some cases, to obtain a detectable signal[24]. Three brain metabolites can currently be identified with proton-MRS: N-acetyl-aspartate, creatine, and choline. It appears, therefore, that MRS is most suitable for the evaluation of biochemical processes occurring in the brain[47], at different steps along the metabolic pathway, that lead to the formation of relatively large amounts of product, even without the administration of exogenous tracer substances.

ET is amenable instead for the assessment of biochemical processes by use of exogenous substances in tracer amounts, when the system studied cannot be perturbed during the study, and when the process examined does not lead to the accumulation of sufficient amounts of product to be measured by MRS. The use of MRS and ET for *in vivo* studies of neurochemistry appears also limited by the poor resolution of both techniques. With respect to the clinical use of these techniques, ET has been widely used for over a decade to assess neurochemical variables useful in the diagnostic work-up of patients with cerebral tumours, cerebrovascular diseases, epilepsy and numerous other pathological states[55]. The potentials of MRS in the examination of the neurological diseases are still largely unexploited[47]. These applications are the object of discussion later in this chapter.

*Pharmacological imaging*

The assessment of neuropharmacological variables can be based on two different strategies. The first requires the administration of pharmacological doses of drugs under investigation and the measurement by imaging techniques, most frequently by ET, of variations of local blood flow or metabolism to define the pattern of functional changes induced by the drug[43]. A second strategy is based on the administration of drugs labelled with radioactive isotopes and the *in vivo* monitoring of the distribution and pharmacokinetics of these tracers[11,79]. In essence, this second strategy allows the *in vivo* definition of the distribution pattern of tracers utilized as specific neuronal markers. This has originated a new form of anatomical imaging and has allowed the visualization in brain of specific populations of neurons that express a specific protein on their surface and thus made it possible to visualize *in vivo* neuronal pathways and projections. ET-based neuropharmacology has subsequently evolved into a methodology based on experimental procedures and kinetic models used in basic biochemical and pharmacological research[12,21,37,81,83]. This methodology is now being applied to measure neuropharmacological variables, such as regional receptor densities, alterations in receptor occupancy from endogenous neurotransmitters and exogenous drugs, and receptor plasticity[49,53,54].

Because of the very low concentration of receptors in brain, their imaging requires the use of tracer substances that once administered in very low amounts to avoid pharmacological effects, can still bind in a concentration that is sufficient to provide an externally detectable signal. This goal can be achieved with ET by the use of tracers with high specific activity (i.e. higher than 1000 Ci/mmol), but it is virtually impossible, at the present time, with MR. The number of radioactively labelled compounds produced for the assessment of several neuropharmacological variables has increased continuously over the last decade since images of brain receptors were produced first with SPET and then with PET[71]. The tracers developed for SPET, all labelled with

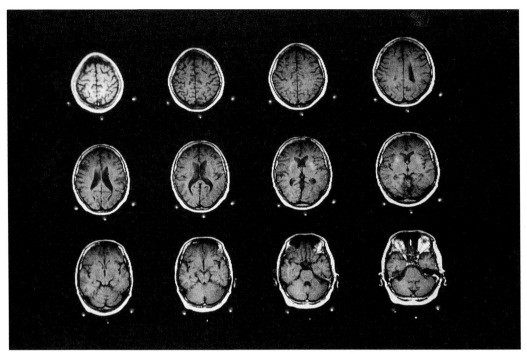

*Fig. 1. Multislice correlation of MRI (black /white scale) and PET/$^{18}$F-fluoroethylspiperone (colour scale) cerebral scans.*

iodine, include substances for the assay of the $D_1$ and $D_2$ dopaminergic receptors, central and peripheral benzodiazepine receptors, $S_1$ and $S_2$ serotoninergic, muscarinic and opiate receptors. Only some of the tracers have been tested also in man, including two highly specific $D_2$ receptor antagonists, IBZM and lisuride, the benzodiazepine antagonist Ro 16-0154 (iomazenil) and the muscarinic antagonist IQNB. Some of these tracers have been used not only for research purposes but also for some clinical applications. Recently, $^{123}$I-CIT has been proposed for the investigation of monoaminergic reuptake sites by SPET. Displacement studies with selective dopaminergic and serotoninergic reuptake inhibitors indicate that this might be useful for the investigation of serotoninergic and dopaminergic innervation in several neurological and psychiatric disorders[71]. Further discussion on neurotransmission and neuroreceptors is given in Chapter 6. However, it is really in the area of PET, rather than SPET, that most of the efforts of the neuropharmacological research with ET have been concentrated. Not only have many of the tracers developed for PET been tested, but they have also been used for the evaluation of patients with neurological and psychiatric disorders. Indeed correct design and application of experimental procedures and kinetic analyses are needed not only to understand basic issues in neuropharmacology, but also to use ET for clinical purposes. Some physiological and pathological processes have been studied in human living subjects only with PET, but not with SPET. PET is at the present unique for quantification of the dynamic processes involved in kinetics (uptake, utilization and excretion) of radioactively labelled chemicals entering the metabolic pathways of the living human being. However, a limited but increasing number of tracers is becoming available also for *in vivo* neurochemistry studies with SPET. These developments will enhance the potentials of SPET as a tool for the *in vivo* visualization of neuronal pathways and projections for the examination of large populations, a goal that appears more suitable for SPET than for PET.

**Imaging of physiological processes**

The localization of functions in the human brain has been based for a long time on the correlation between the *in vivo* observation of neurological and neuropsychological deficits and the detection at autopsy of cerebral lesions. While destructive lesions can cause a functional deficit, irritative lesions are at the basis of pathologically enhanced functions. Both types of lesions have become more identifiable non-invasively *in vivo* by the advent of X-ray CT, MRI and ET. Although the visualization of lesions with X-ray CT or MRI has represented a major event for the *in vivo* explanation of neurological deficits, these systems cannot always be adequate for the full understanding of cerebral function, i.e. processes that require the integrity of neuronal circuits. Thus, the relationship between neuronal activity and cerebral metabolism and haemodynamics has become the basis for studies with PET and SPET of neuronal circuits under resting conditions. Methods for the measurement of blood flow and metabolism during the execution of defined tasks have increased the number of tools available for the assessment of cerebral functional activity[62]. These methods have made possible the definition of neural circuits and pathways involved in sensory-motor activity, attention, memory, word processing, visual recognition. The functional reorganization of human brain after focal injury has been investigated with ET in patients with stroke, and the recruitment of additional motor areas has been reported as well as the reorganization of the brain in different, individual functional patterns. Serial experiments will clarify the temporal dependence of the functional recovery[80]. The use of tracers labelled with short-lived isotopes allows us to perform a complete activation study, i.e. baseline and activation, within the same study session by use of PET, e.g. with $^{15}$O-labelled water or carbon dioxide, or

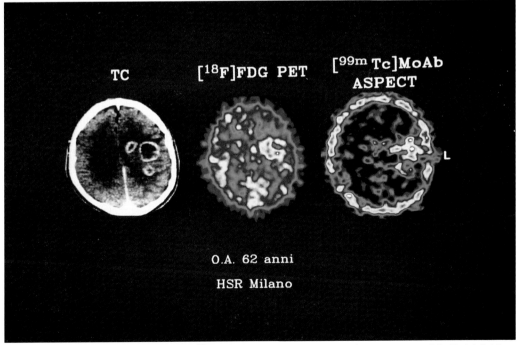

*Fig. 2. Cerebral X-ray CT (left), PET/$^{18}$F-FDG (centre) and SPET with anti-tenascin MoAb (right) images of a patient with glioblastoma of the left frontal lobe. The tumour presents a high metabolic activity in the PET study, and a high tumour/non-tumour activity ratio in the SPECT study performed with the three-step method and biotinylated $^{99m}$Tc-propylamine oxime.*

with radioactive xenon and SPET. The complexity of these techniques and their cost has triggered the development of alternative techniques based on the use of SPET and perfusion tracers (ideally chemical microspheres) labelled with $^{99m}$Tc, and on the performance of the baseline and activation studies at least 24 h apart for the decay of the isotope. A method has recently been validated for motor activation studies that requires the administration of two doses of the tracer, in proportion 1:3, for the baseline and activation study, respectively[59]. However, the best proportion of dose to be administered for optimizing this procedure is not yet well defined .

The recent development of new acquisition procedures and sequences with high temporal resolution, in particular EPI, has made possible the imaging with MRI of physiological processes such as blood microcirculation (perfusion) and the evaluation of molecular mobility (molecular diffusion)[44,45;57]. One area that is specific to MRI is that aimed at the evaluation of molecular diffusion; this area may in the future become of relevance for the assessment of pathological processes such as neoplasms and ischaemia[46]. The use of these techniques has also enabled the monitoring of the transit of a bolus of Gd-DTPA through the cerebral capillary bed; the regional cerebral variation of signal intensity caused by the transit of Gd-DTPA is proportional to the regional blood volume[6]. Visual activation studies showing variations of cerebral blood volume have been performed by this technique[6]. It has also been shown that with MRI changes in tissue contrast, resulting from changes in blood oxygenation, can be detected, deoxygenated blood behaving as an endogenous paramagnetic contrast agent[78]. Based on this feature, changes in cerebral oxygenation have been assessed by fast MRI techniques similar to those observed with ET, with the additional advantage that the artifacts due to the extraparenchymal blood pool observed with ET are partially overcome with these MRI techniques.

Although the results obtained with MRI appear extremely encouraging, in particular for continued progress in the development of instrumentation, the full validation of the results obtained with these techniques, as well as their introduction into a diagnostic process, will require some time.

**Imaging of pathological processes**

The ultimate goal of diagnostic imaging procedures performed in patients with neurological symptoms is the identification of the abnormal morphological and functional patterns that correlate with the symptoms. Thus, methods are evaluated on the basis of their diagnostic sensitivity and specificity. The ideal diagnostic method is rapid, inexpensive, non-invasive and accurate. Currently X-ray CT and MRI are the diagnostic methods of first choice in all neurological diseases[74]. X-ray CT is the technique of first choice for the evaluation of patients in the acute stage following trauma, ischaemic and haemorrhagic stroke, and subarachnoid haemorrhage. MRI is the technique of choice in the subacute and chronic stage of neurological diseases. Both X-ray CT and MRI are very sensitive techniques, but, in numerous cases signs and symptoms cannot be completely explained by methods of morphological imaging. Functional disturbances can, in fact, precede detectable morphological damage; therefore, only functional imaging may permit the early assessment of the biochemical damage that preceds the morphological damage, the correlation of functional alterations and clinical symptoms in the absence of detectable morphological damage, and eventually the explanation of symptoms due to functional abnormalities that occur in areas proximal and remote from the site of the primary lesion, due to diaschisis. Thus, in several cases it is only with the integration of morphological and functional information that it is possible to achieve a full appreciation of the nature and extent of the damage that produces the clinical symptoms. Depending on the disease under examination, its stage, and the question addressed at the time of the observation, the choice of method(s) may vary.

### Cerebrovascular diseases

The non invasive evaluation of patients presenting with cerebrovascular disorders (CVD) by imaging techniques relies mainly on X-ray CT[39]. Other modalities include MRI, SPET perfusion scintigraphy and PET based studies of local haemodynamics and energy metabolism. It has been shown that MRI is superior to X-ray CT for localization of lesions in CVD. One advantage of MRI is that it allows non-invasive angiography[51], useful in the assessment of the cerebral circulation in stroke patients. X-ray CT is used, starting at the time of the stroke onset, for the differential diagnosis between cerebral ischaemia and haemorrhage and for defining the location and size of the lesion. In most cases, however, X-ray CT becomes positive only after several hours of ischaemic stroke. Following the initial diagnostic phase, the sequential examination of stroke patients with X-ray CT or MRI allows the staging of the lesion and helps in the therapeutical planning and follow-up. In the case of transient ischaemic attacks (TIAs) the observation of morphological damage is infrequent, yet possible, as a result of previous ischaemic episodes. During a TIA the defect of perfusion can be demonstrated by a SPET examination. The perfusion defect may persist also after the functional recovery indicating a condition of critical perfusion[8,31]. The non-invasive assessment of other key variables, including the oxygen extraction fraction and metabolism, is only possible with PET[64]. However, PET studies of cerebral haemodynamics and energy metabolism in the acute phase of stroke are not practical in large populations and, for this reason PET cannot be considered a diagnostic tool in these patients[64]. At the time of the stroke onset, therefore, the determination of perfusion by SPET with technetium-labelled tracers may be the only useful measurable variable. The predictive value of SPET perfusion studies on patient outcome and the relation between the results of SPET perfusion studies, X-ray CT, and cerebral angiography has been demonstrated[27]. This observation can have a direct impact on therapeutic planning, one of the most relevant issues in acute stroke patients. The treatment must begin as early as possible, when signs of parenchymal damage are not yet visible with X-ray CT and are of difficult interpretation also with MRI. At this stage of the stroke the assessment by SPET of the extent and severity of the perfusion deficit may be crucial to carry out proper therapy, including therapy with thrombolytic drugs that requires very careful planning due to the attendant risks. The effects of the thrombolytic therapy can be monitored, if necessary, by repeated SPET perfusion studies.

### Brain tumours

For the last two decades the diagnostic work-up of brain tumours has been based on morphological imaging, first with X-ray CT and more recently also with MRI[3,22,28]. Contrast-enhanced X-ray CT is, in general, the first examination performed in patients with a clinical history of brain neoplasm. By use of X-ray CT, it is possible in many cases to make a differential diagnosis with other cerebral lesions and, to a limited extent, also among different types of intracranial tumour. MRI is becoming, however, the primary diagnostic method for its lower negative rate when compared to X-ray CT. X-ray CT and MRI remain largely complementary modalities. In the presence of clinical symptoms leading to the suspicion of tumour, however, negative X-ray CT should be promptly followed by MRI for the detection of possible tumours. X-ray CT remains superior to MRI for the evaluation of bone lesions in proximity of the tumour and calcification within the tumour. The *in vivo* biochemical imaging of tumours is best achieved by emission tomography. The usefulness of FDG in the differentiation between tumour recurrence and radionecrosis has been demonstrated and is widely accepted[14–16]. The possibility of assessing, in sequence, one or more different biochemical and physiological variables of the tumour, including blood flow, oxygen and glucose consumption, protein synthesis, pH, and receptor density, is unique to PET, and this feature may become extremely useful when these measurements are part of defined diagnostic protocols. In the meantime other imaging modalities with SPET and monoclonal antibodies are attracting increasing interest, in particular those aimed at

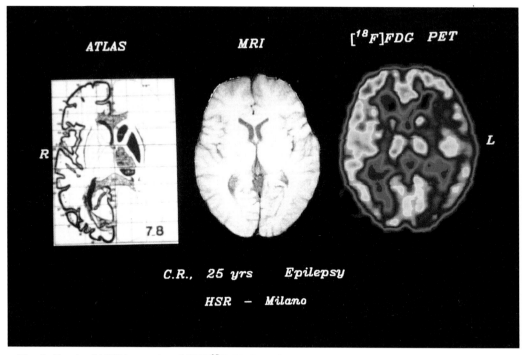

*Fig. 3. Cerebral MRI (centre) and PET/[18]F-FDG (right) images of a patient with refractory epilepsy. Morphological and metabolic images are correlated to the corresponding section of the Talairach & Tournoux[73] atlas (left). A reduction of metabolism in the left temporal and parietal cortex is detected by the PET/[18]F-FDG scan in a morphologically normal area.*

the signal amplification by tumour pre-targeting techniques. This is best achieved with the administration of biotinylated MoAb, followed either by the administration of the radioactive tracer (two-step technique), or by the administration of avidin, after the MoAb, and then by the tracer administration (three-step technique)[58]. The additional steps allow us to achieve a significant signal amplification compared to the single administration of labelled MoAbs. In fact, the binding of the MoAbs to the tumour is a relatively slow biological process compared to the short physical half-life of the radioactive label, thus the separation of the delivery of the MoAb from the radioactive tracer administration allows the use of much smaller doses of radioactivity. By use of biotinylated MoAb and by biotinylation of the carrier of the radioactive tracer, it is possible to enhance further the power of the method. The introduction of an intermediate step, i.e. the administration of avidin, allows first the precipitation of circulating MoAb–avidin complexes that are rapidly eliminated from the bloodstream, i.e. a reduction of the background activity to an acceptable level, and second the enhancement of the binding sites on the tumour. This elegant method is particularly suitable for the investigation of cerebral gliomas with SPET and for differentiating radionecrosis and recurrence; the method has been used for imaging brain tumours within 1 h only of the administration of a [99m]Tc-labelled propyl-amine-oxime-biotin conjugate. However, in principle, the tracer does not need to be a radioactive one and the basic concepts of the method could be transferred to MRI. This procedure, based on the administration of the radioactive tracer only when the tumour is already pretargeted, also opens up interesting perspectives for the treatment of tumours.

By use of MRS, in particular proton-MRS, biochemical variables have been assessed in cerebral

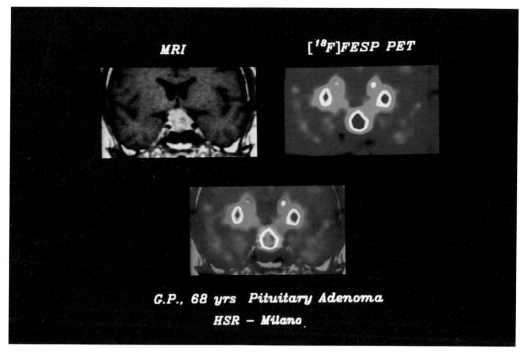

*Fig. 4. Cerebral MRI (top left) and PET/ $^{18}$F-fluoroethylspiperone (top right) images of a patient with a pituitary adenoma. The MRI study defines the morphology of the lesion and of the basal ganglia, while the PET image demonstrates the presence of D2 receptors in the pituitary lesion, as well as in the caudate and the putamen. The two images are overlapped after registration (centre bottom).*

tumours in man. This technique is very sensitive for the detection of derangements from normal metabolism, that are typical of neoplasms. A decrease in the concentration of *N*-acetyl-aspartate is a common finding in cerebral gliomas due to the neuronal concentration of this metabolite exclusively in neurons. Also the presence of a relative increase of choline and lactate characterizes tumours with high metabolic activity. However, despite its high sensitivity, the specificity of proton-MRS in the differentiation of other types of cerebral tumours is relatively poor.

*Epilepsy*

Electrophysiological methods and clinical evaluation are fundamental in the evaluation of patients with seizure disorders. While these procedures are sufficient for the work-up of patients with primary generalized epilepsy, they may not be sufficient to resolve doubts about the cause of seizure and location of the epileptogenic area in patients with partial seizures. Partial epilepsy may be the consequence of a brain lesion, but, in many cases, the assessment of brain morphology with X-ray CT or MRI does not demonstrate a detectable lesion, even though structural alterations below the resolution of the instrumentation may be present (cryptogenetic seizures). In patients with partial seizures the assessment of perfusion and metabolism by ET may allow us to observe areas of interictal hypoperfusion and hypometabolism, and/or increases of perfusion and metabolism during the ictal phase even without evidence of morphological lesions[5,19,75]. For the routine clinical evaluation of patients with epilepsy the combination of interictal and ictal studies of perfusion provide the most complete information[18,63,66]. For this purpose the use of SPET with chemical microspheres is very convenient since it allows us to obtain an image of the

143

perfusion at the time of the tracer injection, i.e. during seizures, by performing the SPET study at the end of the seizures. Assessment of perfusion and metabolism is used by some surgeons in the presurgical evaluation of patients with medically refractory partial epilepsy to confirm the uniqueness of the focus and its location. This practice, however, has not yet gained widespread acceptance and is considered in many cases insufficient for surgical intervention without stereo-EEG with depth electrodes. PET and SPET studies in epileptic patients have shown that the area of altered flow and metabolism is often wider than the epileptogenic zone and that there are within the hypometabolic and underperfused areas various zones with different electrical activity: epileptogenic, irritative, and lesional[30]. Thus the relation between electrical activity and perfusion/metabolic alterations needs further clarification in order to achieve a full exploitation of the SPET and PET information in planning the surgical therapy. Recently a high sensitivity of proton-MRI and proton-MRS imaging (chemical shift imaging) in the detection of both the location and extension of the epileptic focus in patients with intractable temporal lobe epilepsy has been demonstrated[52]. These MR methods, however, are still under evaluation.

## Dementia

In dementia-associated disorders the diagnosis is usually based on clinical evaluation and can only be proved by neuropathological examination. In a number of cases, however, the clinical diagnosis is questionable, in particular in the early stages of Alzheimer's disease (AD), and additional information is often sought from neuroimaging techniques[23]. X-ray CT and MRI may contribute to the definition of the presence and degree of cerebral atrophy or cerebral lesions (e.g. cerebrovascular disorders, hydrocephalus, subdural haematoma or tumours) that may in some cases determine the occurrence of cognitive impairment similar to what is observed in dementia. However, the use of methods of morphological imaging may often be inconclusive for the diagnosis of dementia, since the atrophy that can be observed is not specific to the disease; in a large number of patients the X-ray examination demonstrates the presence of atrophy of variable degree, focal or diffuse to the whole brain, usually unrelated to the neurological and neuropsychological symptoms presented by the patients. In some cases also the presence of periventricular and deep white matter abnormalities can be observed with MRI, but the demonstration of these lesions is not sufficient to explain the neurological deficits. MRI studies performed to examine selectively specific brain structures, i.e. the hippocampus, may eventually be more conclusive and useful in the evaluation of patients with AD. The assessment of cerebral metabolism and blood flow with ET has been shown to be useful in the evaluation of demented patients, particularly in the early phase of probable Alzheimer's disease. A pattern of bilateral hypometabolism has been consistently demonstrated in the parietal and temporal cortex[1,34,42]. However, the use of PET studies has recently been questioned since also other patterns of altered perfusion and metabolism have been observed in dementia, including hypometabolism of the frontal cortex[17] as well as an asymmetric cortical hypometabolism, mainly in the early phase of AD[33,48,56,65]. Moreover the temporo-parietal hypometabolism cannot be considered specific to AD. Nonetheless, the presence of the hypometabolic temporo-parietal pattern has a high prognostic value for the development of AD.

In parallel with PET studies, a reduction of perfusion in the temporal and parietal areas, in patients with AD, has been shown also by SPET[10,25,38,40,61]. The ability of SPET, used in combination with blood flow tracers, to separate patients with dementia from normal elderly controls has also been reported to be high: 86 per cent[13]. We have recently carried out a systematic comparison of the sensitivity of PET and SPET techniques in the same series of patients with AD (Messa et al., in press) by a dedicated SPET machine[26] and $^{99m}$Tc-HMPAO, significant differences between AD patients and controls were found both with PET and CER-ASPECT in the parietal and temporal cortices, and differences were inconsistently observed only in other associative areas.

## Summary

Methods of structural and functional imaging, i.e. X-ray CT, MRI, and emission tomography (ET), have considerable impact on the diagnostic work-up, staging, therapeutic planning, interventional therapy, and follow-up of patients. The same methods can also be used for the examination of issues in biochemistry, pharmacology, and physiology. The information acquired with the various imaging modalities is often complementary, and thus the synergistic and integrated use of two or more imaging modalities to gain new insight on the status and function of an organ is becoming increasingly important. The synergistic approach can yield new information with little extra acquisition cost; it could, therefore, become the basis for the modification of current diagnostic procedures. This paper summarizes the advancement and application of synergistic use of biomedical imaging technologies (BITs) in the following areas:

(1) Technological: instrumentation, development and production of radiotracers, image registration;

(2) Clinical: application of the synergistic use of BITs in diagnostic protocols;

(3) Research: application of different BITS for pharmacological, neurochemical and physiological research.

The ultimate goal of synergistic brain imaging is the optimization of clinical protocols to incorporate the knowledge gained by the use of different BITs. The technological aspects are preliminary and essential for the development and application of BITs for physiological research and clinical application. The integration of basic research and informatics with clinical applications must be sought, in order to develop a new strategy designed to provide clinicians with results obtained from the integrated use of BITs rather than fragmented individual diagnostic reports.

## *Acknowledgements*

The authors wish to thank K. Schmidt for useful discussion, M. Belloli and L. Scarda for their secretarial help. This project has been partially financed by CNR Progetto Finalizzato Invecchiamento INV93–2–280.

## References

1. Alavi, A., Dann, R., Chawluk, J., Alavi, J., Kushner, M. & Reivich, M. (1986): Positron emission tomography imaging of regional cerebral glucose metabolism. *Semin. Nucl. Med.* **16**, 2–34.

2. Arun, K.S., Huang T.S. & Blostein S.D. (1987): Least-squares fitting of two 3-D point sets. *IEEE Trans. PAMI* **9**, 698–700.

3. Atlas, S.W. (1991): Intraaxial brain tumours. In: *Magnetic resonance imaging of the brain and spine*, ed. S. W. Atlas, pp. 379–409. New York: Raven Press.

4. Bailey, D., Jones, T., Spinks, T.J., Gilardi, M.C. & Townsend, D.W. (1991): Noise equivalent count measurements in a neuro-PET scanner with retractable septa. *IEEE Trans. Med. Imag.* **10**, 256–260.

5. Baldy-Moulinier, M., Lassen, N.A., Engel, J. & Askienazy, S. (1989): eds. *Focal epilepsy; clinical use of emission tomography.* London, Paris, Rome: John Libbey.

6. Belliveau, J.W., Kennedy, D.N., McKinstry, R.C., Buchbinder, B.R., Weisskoff, R.M., Cohen, M.S., Vevea, J.M., Brady, T.J. & Rosen, B.R. (1991): Functional mapping of the human visual cortex by magnetic resonance imaging. *Science* **254**, 716–719.

7. Bettinardi, V., Scardaoni, R., Gilardi, M.C., Rizzo, G., Perani, D., Paulesu, E., Striano, G., Triulzi, F. & Fazio, F. (1991): A new head-holder for patient positioning repositioning and fixation in PET, MR and CT devices. *J. Comput. Assist. Tomogr.* **15**, 886–892.

8. Bogousslawsky, J., Delaloye-Bishof, A., Regli, F. & Delaloye, B. (1990): Prolonged hypoperfusion and early stroke after transient ischaemic attack. *Stroke* **21**, 40–46

145

9.    Budinger, T.J. (1990): Advances in emission tomography. *J. Nucl. Med.* **31**, 628–631.

10.   Burns, A., Philpot, M.P., Costa, D.C., Ell, P.J. & Levy, R. (1989): The investigation of Alzheimer's disease with single photon emission tomography. *J. Neurol. Neurosur. Psychiatry* **52**, 248–253.

11.   Comar, D., Mazière, M., Godot, J.M., Berger, G., Soussaline, F., Menini, C., Arfel, G. & Naquet, R. (1979): Visualization of [11]C-flunitrazepam displacement in the brain of the live baboon. *Nature* **280**, 329–331.

12.   Delforge, J., Syrota, A. & Mazoyer, B.M. (1990): Identifiability analysis and parameter identification of an *in vivo* ligand-receptor model from PET data. *IEEE Trans. Biomed. Eng.* **37**, 653–662.

13.   Dewan, M., & Gupta, S. (1992): Toward a definite diagnosis of Alzheimer's disease. *Compr. Psychiatry* **33**, 282–290.

14.   Di Chiro, G., De LaPaz, R.L., Brooks, R.A., Sokoloff, L., Kornblith, P.L.,, Smith, B.H., Patronas, N.J., Kufta, C.V., Kessler, R.M., Johnson, G.S., Manning, R.G. & Wolf, A.P. (1982): Glucose utilization of cerebral gliomas measured by [18]F-fluorodeoxyglucose and positron emission tomography. *Neurology* **32**, 1323–1329.

15.   Di Chiro, G. & Brooks, R.A. (1988): PET-FDG of untreated and treated cerebral gliomas. *J. Nucl. Med.* **29**, 421–422.

16.   Di Chiro, G., Oldfield, E., Wright, D.C., De Michele, G., Patronas, N., Doppman, J.L., Larson, S.M., Masanori, Ito & Kufta, C.V. (1988): Cerebral necrosis after radiotherapy and/or intraarterial chemotherapy for brain tumours, PET and neuropathologic studies. *Am. J. Roentg.* **150**, 189–197.

17.   Duara, R., Grady, C., Haxby, J., Sundaram, M., Cutler, N.R., Heston, L., Moore, A., Sclageter, N., Larson, S. & Rapoport, S.I. (1986): Positron emission tomography in Alzheimer's disease. *Neurology* **36**, 879–887.

18.   Duncan, R., Bone, I., Patterson, J. & Hadley, D.M. (1989): SPECT in temporal lobe epilepsy: interictal and postictal studies. In: *Current problems in epilepsy (7). Focal epilepsy: clinical use of emission tomography,* eds. M. Baldy-Moulinier, N.A. Lassen, J. Engel Jr, S. Askienazy, pp. 79–96. London, Paris, Rome: John Libbey.

19.   Engel, J. (1988): The role of neuroimaging in the surgical treatment of epilepsy. *Acta Neurol. Scand.* **45**, 84–89.

20.   Evans, A.C., Marrett, S., Collins, L. & Peters, T.M. (1989): Anatomical functional correlative analysis of the human brain using three dimensional imaging system. *SPIE 1092 Medical Imaging* **111**, Image processing, 264–274.

21.   Farde, L., Halldin, C., Stone-Elander, S. & Sedvall, G. (1987): PET analysis of human dopamine receptor subtypes using [1]C-SCH 23390 and [11]C-raclopride. *Psychopharmacology* **92**, 278–284.

22.   Fishbein, D.S. (1988): Neuroradiologic work-up of brain tumours. In: *Clinical neuroimaging*, ed. W.H. Theodore, pp. 111–137. New York: Alan R. Liss.

23.   Friedland, R.P. & Luxenberg, J. (1988): Neuroimaging and dementia. In: *Clinical neuroimaging*, ed. W.H. Theodore, pp. 139–163. New York: Alan R. Liss.

24.   Gadian, D.G. (1982): *Nuclear magnetic resonance and its applications to living systems.* Oxford: Clarendon Press.

25.   Gemmel, H.G., Sharp, P.F., Smith, F.W., Besson, J., Ebmeier, K., Davidson, J. *et al.* (1989): Cerebral blood flow measured by SPECT as a diagnostic tool in the study of dementia. *Psychiatry Res.* **29**, 327–329.

26.   Genna, S. & Smith, A.P. (1988): The development of ASPECT, an annular single crystal brain camera for high efficiency SPECT. *IEEE Trans. Nucl. Sci.* **35**, 654–658.

27.   Giubilei, F., Lenzi, G.L., Di Piero, V., Pozzili, C., Pantano, P., Bastianello, S., Argentino, C. & Fieschi, C. (1990): Predictive value of brain perfusion single-photon emission computed tomography in acute ischaemic stroke. *Stroke* **21**, 895–900.

28.   Goldberg, H.I. (1991): Extraaxial brain tumours. In: *Magnetic resonance imaging of the brain and spine.* ed. S. W. Atlas, pp. 327–377. New York: Raven Press.

29.   Gore, J.C. (1991): Contrast agents and relaxation effects. In: *Magnetic resonance imaging of the brain and spine.* ed. S. W. Atlas, pp. 69–85. New York: Raven Press.

30.   Habert, M.O., Parietti, L., Lebtahi, R., Piketty, M.L., Tassi, L., Mary, R., Broglin, D., Askienazy, S. & Munari, C. (1989): A [99m]Tc-HmPAO interictal study in severe partial epilepsies: correlations with anatomical and electrophysiological data. In: *Current problems in epilepsy (7). Focal epilepsy; clinical use of emission tomography* eds. M. Baldy-Moulinier, N.A. Lassen, J. Engel Jr, S. Askienazy, pp. 197–209. London, Paris, Rome: John Libbey.

31.   Hartmann, A. (1985): Prolonged disturbances of regional cerebral blood flow in transient ischaemic attacks. *Stroke* **16**, 932–939.

32. Hawkes, D.J., Hill, D.L.G., Lehmann, E.D., Robinson, G.P., Maisey, M.N. & Colchester, A.C.F. (1990): Preliminary work on the interpretation of SPECT images with the aid of registered MR images and an MR derived 3D neuro-anatomical atlas. *NATO ASI Series* **F60**, 241–251.

33. Haxby, J.V., Duara, R., Grady, C.L., Cutler, N.R. & Rapoport, S.I. (1985): Relations between neuropsychological and cerebral metabolic asymmetries in early Alzheimer's disease. *J. Cereb. Blood Flow Metab.* **5**, 193–200.

34. Haxby, J.V., Grady, C.L., Duara, R., Sclageter, N., Berg, G. & Rapoport, S.I. (1986): Neocortical metabolic abnormalities precede nonmemory cognitive defects in early Alzheimer's type dementia. *Arch. Neurol.* **43**, 882–885.

35. Hoffman, E.J. & Phelps, M.E. (1986): Positron emission tomography principles and quantitation. In: *Positron emission tomography and autoradiography: principles and application for the brain and heart,* eds. M. Phelps, J. Mazziotta & H. Schelbert, pp. 237–286. New York: Raven Press.

36. Huang S.C. & Phelps, M.E. (1986): Principles of tracer kinetic modeling in positron emission tomography and autoradiography. In: *Positron emission tomography and autoradiography: principles and application for the brain and heart,* eds. M. Phelps, J Mazziotta & H. Schelbert, pp. 287–346. New York: Raven Press.

37. Huang, S.C., Bahn, M.M., Barrio, J.R., Hoffman, J.M., Satyamurthy, N., Hawkins, R.A., Mazziotta, J.C. & Phelps, M.E. (1989): A double-injection technique for *in vivo* measurement of dopamine $D_2$-receptor density in monkeys with 3-(2'-[18]F)fluoro-ethyl-spiperone and dynamic positron emission tomography. *J. Cereb. Blood Flow Metab.* **9**, 850–858.

38. Jagust, A.J., Budinger, T.F. & Reed, B.R. (1987): The diagnosis of dementia with single photon emission computed tomography. *Arch. Neurol.* **44**, 258–262.

39. Jarenwattananon, A., Khandji, A. & Brust, J.C.M. (1988): Diagnostic neuroimaging in stroke. In: *Clinical neuroimaging,* ed. W.H. Theodore, pp. 11–47. New York: Alan R. Liss.

40. Johnson, K.A., Mueller, S.T., Walsche, T.M., English, R.J. & Holman, B.L. (1987): Cerebral perfusion imaging in Alzheimer's disease: use of single photon emission computed tomography and lofetamine hydrochloride [123]I. *Arch. Neurol.* **44**,165–168.

41. Kouris, K., Jarritt, P.H., Costa, D.C. & Ell, P.J. (1992): Physical assessment of the GE/CGR Neurocam and comparison with a single rotating gamma-camera. *Eur. J. Nucl. Med.* **19**, 236–242.

42. Kuhl, D.E., Small, G.W., Riege, W.H., Fujikawa, E.J., Metter, E.J., Benson, D.E., Ashford, J.W., Mazziotta, J.C., Maltese, A. & Dorsey, D.A. (1987): Cerebral metabolic patterns before the diagnosis of probable Alzheimer's disease. *J. Cereb. Blood Flow Metab.* **7**, S406.

43. Kurumaji, A., Dewar, D. & McCulloch, J. (1993): Metabolic mapping with deoxyglucose autoradiography as an approach for assessing drug action in the central nervous system. In: *Imaging drug action in the brain,* ed. E.D. London, pp. 207–246. USA: CRC Press.

44. Le Bihan, D. (1991): Molecular diffusion nuclear resonance imaging. *Mag. Res. Quart.* **7**, 1–30.

45. Le Bihan, D., Turner, R., Moonen, C.T. & Pekar, J. (1991): Imaging of diffusion and microcirculation with gradient sensitization: design, strategy, and significance. *J. Mag. Res. Imag.* **1**, 7–28.

46. Le Bihan, D., Turner, R., Douek, P. & Patronas, N. (1991): Diffusion MR imaging: clinical applications. *Am. J. Roentg.* **159**, 591–599.

47. Lenkinski, R.E.& Schnall, M.D. (1991): MR spectroscopy and the biochemical basis of neurological disease. In: *Magnetic resonance imaging of the brain and spine,* ed. S. W. Atlas, pp. 1099–1121. New York: Raven Press.

48. Loewenstein, D., Yoshii, F., Barker, W.W., Apicella, A., Emran, A., Chang, J.Y. & Duara, R. (1987): Predominant left hemispheric metabolic deficit predicts early manifestation of dementia. *J. Cereb. Blood Flow Metab.* **7**, S416.

49. Lucignani, G., Moresco, R.M. & Fazio, F. (1989): PET-based neuropharmacology: state of the art. *Cerebrovasc. Brain Metab. Rev.* **1**, 271–287.

50. Mandava, V. R., Fitzpatrick, J. M., Maurer, C.R. Jr., Maciunas, R.J. & Allen, G.S. (1992): Registration of multimodal volume head images via attached markers. *SPIE, 1652 Medical Imaging VI: Image processing,* 271'–282.

51. Masaryk, T.J. & Ross, J.S. (1991): MR angiography: clinical applications. In: *Magnetic resonance imaging of the brain and spine,* ed. S. W. Atlas, pp. 1079–1097. New York: Raven Press.

52.  Matthews, P.M., Andermann, F. & Arnold, D.L. (1990): A proton magnetic resonance spectroscopy study of focal epilepsy in humans. *Neurology* **40**, 985–989.

53.  Mazière, B. & Mazière, M. (1990): Where have we got to with neuroreceptor mapping of the human brain? *Eur. J. Nucl. Med.* **16**, 817–835.

54.  Mazière, B. & Mazière, M. (1991): Positron emission tomography studies of brain receptors. *Fundam. Clin. Pharmacol.* **5**, 61–91.

55.  Mazziotta, J.C. & Phelps, M.E. (1986): Positron emission tomography studies of the brain. In: *Positron emission tomography and autoradiography: principles and application for the brain and heart*, eds. M. Phelps, J. Mazziotta & H. Schelbert, pp. 493–579. New York: Raven Press.

56.  McGeer, P.L., Kamo, H., Harrop., R., Li, D.K.B., Tuokko, H., McGeer, E.G., Adam, M.J., Ammann, W., Beattie, B.L., Clane, D.B., Martin, W.R.W., Pate, B.D., Rogers, J.G., Ruth, T.J., Sayre, C. & Stoessel, A.J. (1986): Positron emission tomography in patients with clinically diagnosed Alzheimer's disease. *Can. Med. Assoc. J.* **134**, 597–607.

57.  Ogawa, S., Lee, T.-M., Nayak, A.S. & Glynn, P. (1990): Oxygenation-sensitive contrast in magnetic resonance image of rodent brain at high magnetic fields. *Magn. Res. Med.* **14**, 68–78.

58.  Paganelli, G., Magnani, P., Zito, F., Villa, E., Stella, M., Lopalco, L., Siccardi, A.G. & Fazio, F. (1991). Antibody guided tumour detection in CEA positive patients using the avidin-biotin system. *Cancer Res.* **51**, 5960–5966.

59.  Pantano, P., Di Piero, V., Ricci, M., Fieschi, C., Bozzao, L. & Lenzi, G.L. (1992): Motor stimulation response by technetium-99m hexamethylpropylene amine oxime split-dose method and single photon emission tomography. *Eur. J. Nucl. Med.* **19**, 939–945.

60.  Pelizzari, C.A., Chen, G.T.Y., Spelbring, D.R., Weichselbraum, R.R. & Chen, C.T. (1989): Accurate three-dimensional registration of CT, PET and/or MR images of the brain. *J. Comput. Assist. Tomogr.* **13**, 20–26

61.  Perani, D., Di Piero, V., Vallar, G., Cappa, S., Messa, C., Bottini, G., Berti, A., Passafiume, D., Scarlato, G., Gerundini, P., Lenzi, G.L. & Fazio, F. (1988): Tc-99m-HMPAO-SPECT study of regional cerebral perfusion in early Alzheimer's disease. *J. Nucl. Med.* **29**, 1507–1514.

62.  Perani, D., Gilardi, M.C., Cappa, S.F. & Fazio, F. (1993): PET studies of cognitive functions: a review. *J. Nucl. Med. Biol.* **36**, 324–336.

63.  Podreka, I., Lang, W., Mayr, N., Goldenberg, G., Schmidbauer, M., Topitz, A., Steiner, M., Müller, Ch., Brücke, Th., Asenbaum, S. & Deecke, L. (1989): Ictal and postictal HmPAO-SPECT studies in patients suffering from partial complex seizures. In: *Current problems in epilepsy (7). Focal epilepsy; clinical use of emission tomography*, eds. M. Baldy-Moulinier, N.A. Lassen, J. Engel Jr & S. Askienazy, pp. 167–175. London, Paris, Rome: John Libbey.

64.  Powers, W.J. (1988): Positron emission tomography in cerebrovascular disease: clinical applications? In: *Clinical neuroimaging*, ed. W.H. Theodore, pp. 11–47. New York: Alan R. Liss.

65.  Powers, W.J., Perlmutter, J.S., Videen, T.O., Herscovitch, P., Griffeth, L.K., Royal, H.D., Siegel, B.A., Morris, J.C. & Berg, L. (1992): Blinded clinical evaluation of positron emission tomography for diagnosis of probable Alzheimer's disease. *Neurology* **42**, 765–770.

66.  Rowe, C.C., Berkovic, F., Benjamin Sia, S.T., Austin, M., McKay, J.W., Kalnins, R.M. & Bladin, P. (1989): Localization of epileptic foci with postictal single photon emission computed tomography. *Ann. Neurol.* **26**, 660–668.

67.  Schmidt, K., Lucignani, G., Moresco, R.M., Rizzo, G., Gilardi, M.C., Messa, C., Colombo, C., Fazio, F. & Sokoloff, L. (1992): Errors introduced by tissue heterogeneity in estimation of local cerebral glucose utilization with current kinetic models of the $^{18}$F-fluorodeoxyglucose method. *J. Cereb. Blood Flow Metab.* **12**, 823–834.

68.  Shellock, F.G. (1991): Bioeffects and safety considerations. In: *Magnetic resonance imaging of the brain and spine*, ed. S. W. Atlas, pp. 87–107. New York: Raven Press.

69.  Sokoloff, L. (1986): Cerebral circulation, energy metabolism, and protein synthesis: general characteristics and principles of measurement. In: *Positron emission tomography and autoradiography: principles and application for the brain and heart*, eds. M. Phelps, J. Mazziotta & H. Schelbert, pp. 1–71. New York: Raven Press.

70.  Spinks, T.J., Jones, T., Bailey, D.L. & Towsend, D.W., Grootoonk, S., Bloomfield, P.M., Gilardi, M.C., Casey, M.E., Sipe, B. & Reed, J. (1992): Physical performance of a positron tomograph for brain imaging with retractable septa. *Phys. Med. Biol.* **37**, 1637–1655.

71.  Stocklin, G. (1992): Tracers for metabolic imaging of brain and heart. *Eur. J. Nucl. Med.* **19**, 527–551.

72.    Stehling, M.K., Turner, R. & Mansfield, P. (1991): Echo-planar imaging, magnetic resonance imaging in a fraction of a second. *Science* **254**, 43–54.

73.    Talairach, J. & Tournoux, P. (1988): *Co-planar stereotactic atlas of the human brain: 3-dimensional proportional system: an approach to cerebral imaging.* Stuttgart, New York: G.T. Verlag.

74.    Theodore, W. H. (1988): ed. *Clinical neuroimaging.* New York: Alan R. Liss.

75.    Theodore, W. H. (1988): Epilepsy. In: *Clinical neuroimaging,* ed. W.H. Theodore, pp. 183–210. New York: Alan R. Liss.

76.    Tofts, P. & Wray, S. (1988): A critical assessment of methods of measuring metabolite concentrations by NMR spectroscopy. *NMR Biomed.* **1**, 1-10.

77.    Townsend, D.W., Geissbuhler, A., Defrise, M., Hoffman, E.J., Spinks, T.J., Bailey, D.L., Gilardi, M.C. & Jones, T. (1991): Fully three dimensional reconstruction for a PET camera with retractable septa. *IEEE Trans. Med. Imag.* **10**, 505–512.

78.    Turner, R., Le Bihan, D., Moonen, C.T., Despres, D. & Frank, J. (1991): Echo-planar time course of MRI cat brain oxygenation changes. *Magn. Res. Med.* **22**, 159–166.

79.    Wagner, H.N., Burns, H.D., Dannals, R.F. *et al.* (1983): Imaging dopamine receptors in the human brain by positron tomography. *Science* **221**, 1264–1266.

80.    Weiller, C., Ramsay, S.C., Wise, R.J.S., Friston, K.J. & Frackowiak, R.S.J. (1993): Individual patterns of functional reorganization in the human cerebral cortex after capsular infarction. *Ann. Neurol.* **33**, 181–189.

81.    Wong, D.F., Wagner, H.N., Dannals, R.F., Links, J.M., Frost, J.H.J., Ravert, H.T., Wilson, A.A., Rosenbaum, A.E., Gjedde, A., Douglass, K.H., Petronis, J.D., Folstein, M.F., Toung, J.K.T., Burns, H.D. & Kuhar, M.D. (1984): Effects of age on dopamine and serotonin receptors measured by positron tomography in the living human brain. *Science* **226**, 1393–1396.

82.    Woods, R. P., Cherry, S.R. & Mazziotta, J.C. (1992): Rapid automated algorithm for aligning and reslicing PET images. *J. Comput. Assist. Tomogr.* **16**, 620–633.

83.    Young, A.B., Frey, K.A. & Agranoff B.W. (1986): Receptor assays *in vitro* and *in vivo.* In: *Positron emission tomography and autoradiography: principles and application for the brain and heart* eds. M. Phelps, J. Mazziotta & H. Schelbert, pp. 73–111. New York: Raven Press.

# *APPENDIX*

# Appendix

This final section illustrates some of the patterns one is likely to find in the clinical routine application of brain perfusion imaging with SPET and contains a few examples of characteristic appearances of neuroreceptor SPET studies. First of all, the regional distribution of a brain perfusion radiotracer is described in comparison with the anatomical relationship between structures of well known and distinct brain–blood flow (rCBF) rates in the normal man. The column on the left hand side of plate A1 shows drawings of the regional intracerebral anatomy from the level of the cerebellum (on the bottom) to the superior frontal and parietal lobes sliced through the periventricular white matter (on the top). The colour images on the right hand side display the distribution of the regional brain perfusion SPET patterns with similar orientation and at identical planes to the anatomical references. The small insert illustrates the level of each pair of horizontal slices with reference to the surface of the left hemisphere.

The colour scale bar is included for a quick semi-quantitative assessment of the perfusion patterns once all the slices are scaled to the maximum counts per pixel in the entire study, most frequently found in the cerebellum of normal individuals, when no stimulation paradigm has been used either before or during the injection. In summary, black is ascribed to the background and yellow and white to the pixels (structures) with higher brain perfusion values (e.g. cerebellum, visual cortex/calcarine gyrus and basal ganglia, with an almost 1:1 relationship). The remainder of this 16 step non-linear colour scale helps to find differences between all the other structures with distinct regional brain perfusion values. Cerebellum, vermis, midbrain (brain stem including pons), temporal lobes, visual cortex (calcarine gyrus), thalamus, caudate nucleus, putamen/globus pallidus, cingulate gyrus, corpus callosum, lateral ventricles, paraventricular white matter, and grey matter of frontal, parietal and occipital cortices are labelled amongst other structures for easy reference.

The majority of colour figures in this appendix will display this colour scheme. However, some cases will be shown with a linear black and white colour scale (B&W) for the benefit of those who prefer B&W rather than a non-linear scale.

ACKNOWLEDGEMENTS
Image A14 is courtesy of M.D. Devous, Dept of Nuclear Medicine, University of Texas Southwestern Medical Center, Dallas, Texas, USA. Images on example A15 were obtained at the Department of Nuclear Medicine, Charing Cross Hospital, London, UK, and images on examples A20 and A21 are from ongoing collaborative work with Dr L. Pilowsky, Institute of Psychiatry, London, UK. All the other examples are from the Institute of Nuclear Medicine, UCL Medical School, London, UK.)

# Normal

## *Example A1*

Comparison between anatomy and regional brain perfusion in normal man. The images in the right column are horizontal slices from the SPET study of a 40-year-old normal male.

bs = brainstem; c = cerebellum; cg = cyngulate gyrus; cn = caudate nucleus; fc = frontal cortex; ifc = inferior frontal cortex; lv = lateral ventricle; pc = parietal cortex; th = thalamus; tc = temporal cortex; tlc = lateral cortex of the temporal lobe; tmc = medial cortex of the temporal lobe; v = vermis; vc = visual cortex; wm = white matter

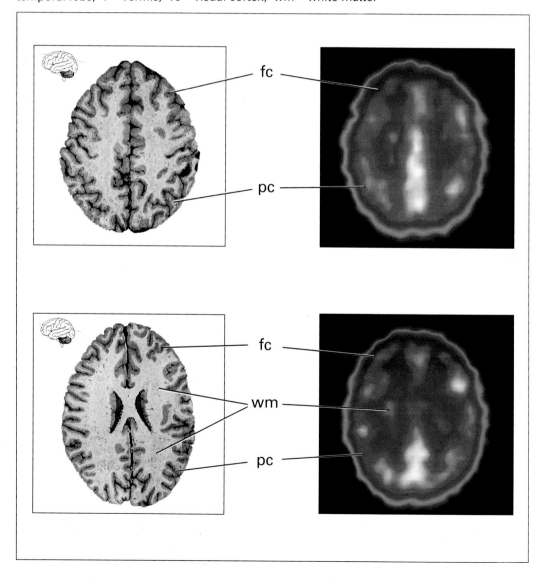

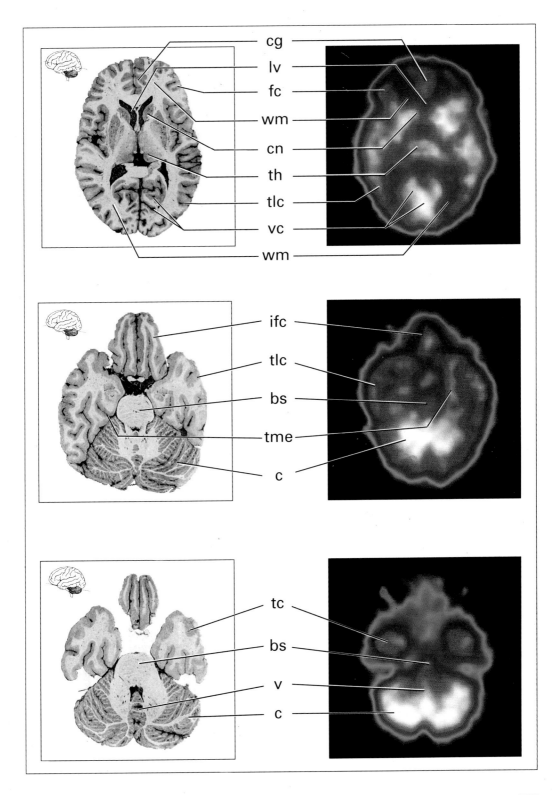

# Normal

### Example A2

*Description* – Although in the first example only horizontal slices were shown for the comparison with the intracerebral brain structures, it must be emphasized that the three main orientation SPET slices (sagittal and coronal in addition to horizontal) should be studied on every patient investigation. *Transverse or horizontal* slices are parallel to the AC–PC (anterior comissure – posterior comissure) line. This line is difficult to identify on SPET brain perfusion images. However, if one joins the inferior frontal cortex with the inferior area of the occipital cortex on a sagittal slice, a plane parallel to the AC–PC line is defined as reference for the transverse/horizontal slices. *Coronal slices* are perpendicular to the horizontal ones and enable simultaneous displays of temporal and parietal cortices. In addition, they show both the medial and lateral, as well as the inferior, cortex on every slice through the temporal lobes. *Sagittal* slices are parallel to the plane containing the interhemispheric groove and the longitudinal midsection of the third ventricle. They are ideal to compare frontal with parietal cortices on the same paramedial slice.

The example shows in B&W the distribution of brain perfusion patterns on a SPET study from a 35-year-old normal male.

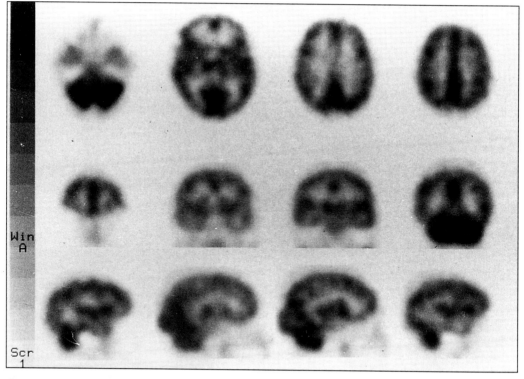

*Comments*

- Normal regional brain perfusion on young people demonstrate higher values to the cerebellum and primary visual cortex.

  With the present state of the art SPET spatial and contrast resolution it is not possible to distinguish white matter from ventricles.

# Normal

## *Example A3*

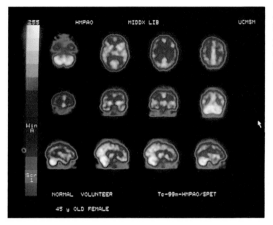

*Description* – Distribution of regional brain perfusion rates on a SPET study from a 45-year-old normal female. There are no significant asymmetries on the distribution of the radiotracer throughout the different brain structures, either cortical or subcortical.

## *Example A4*

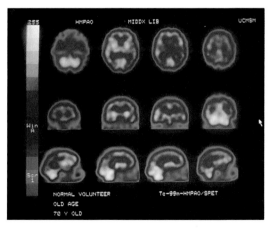

*Description* – Distribution of regional perfusion rates on a SPET study from a 70-year-old normal male. The low perfusion space lying between the head of the caudate nuclei appears larger than in the studies from young normals. Small cortical asymmetries, particularly fronto-parietal, are seen. These are now considered to be a characteristic feature of SPET studies of normal ageing.

*Comments*

- There is a global decrease in glucose metabolism and cerebral blood flow with age. However, interhemispheric asymmetries of regional blood flow and perfusion values seem to be more characteristic and significant on elderly than young normal volunteers. Care must be taken when interpreting brain perfusion SPET studies of elderly populations.

  Normal databases are more and more necessary for adequate semi-quantification. Ideally, the presently available methodology for quantification of rCBF with perfusion tracers should be further developed and validated.

# Dementia of the Alzheimer type (DAT)

### Example A5

*Description* – This brain perfusion SPET study from an 80-year-old male with advanced DAT demonstrates bilateral and almost symmetrical reduction of the regional perfusion rates in the temporal, parietal and frontal cortices. In addition there is enlargement of the space between the head of the caudate nuclei, indicative of ventricular dilatation.

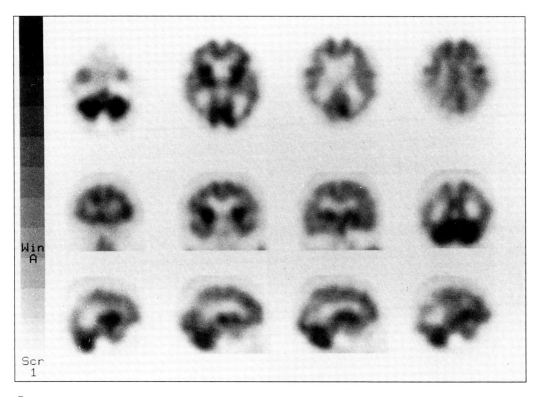

*Comment*

- Although there is no report to date showing a consistent pattern of brain perfusion abnormalities in DAT, this bilateral and almost symmetrical decrease of the regional perfusion rates to the temporal and parietal cortices supports the clinical diagnosis of DAT. In advanced cases, involvement of frontal cortex will be observed.

# Dementia of the Alzheimer type (DAT)

## *Example A6*

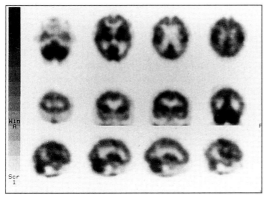

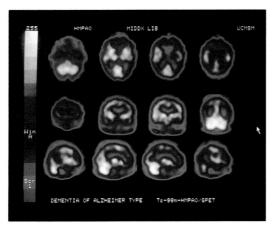

*Description* – The images show a comparison between B&W and colour display of the same brain perfusion SPET study of a 69-year-old male with DAT. There is bilateral reduction of the regional perfusion rates, symmetrical on the parietal cortex, and distinctly asymmetrical on the temporal (lower on the left) and frontal (lower on the right) cortices. Regional perfusion to visual cortex, basal ganglia and fronto-parietal motor cortex on both hemispheres is preserved. The cerebellum appears symmetrical and within normal limits.

## *Comments*

• SPET studies in patients with DAT show bilateral (either symmetrical or asymmetrical) reduction of the regional brain perfusion values in the temporal and parietal cortices, with involvement of the frontal cortex in the more advanced states of the disease. Ventricular dilatation may be seen due to enlargement of the space between the head of the caudate nuclei.

# Dementia with multiple infarcts (MID)

### Example A7

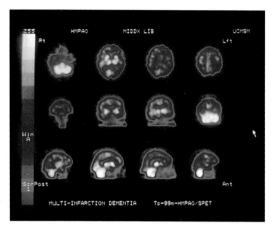

*Description* – This brain perfusion SPET study from a 72-year-old male with MID demonstrates characteristic wedge-shaped perfusion deficits (almost triangular in shape) in the left frontal cortex, right and left parietal cortices and left temporal lobe. They are not symmetrical either on intensity of uptake or anatomical distribution. They originate clear-cut deficits on the cortical boundary, on opposition to the reduction (not wedge-shaped) of brain perfusion seen in patients with DAT.

### Example A8

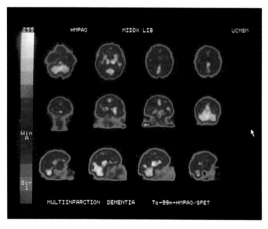

*Description* – This brain perfusion SPET study from a 76-year-old female with MID demonstrates small perfusion deficits in the right and left frontal and parietal cortices, with almost preserved perfusion rates to the temporal lobes. The small perfusion deficits are not symmetrical in size or localization. There is slightly lower perfusion to the basal ganglia compared to normal, and the distribution of the regional perfusion values is more irregular than in patients with DAT.

*Comments*

- SPET studies in patients with MID frequently show irregular distribution of the radiotracer (regional brain perfusion rates) with wedge-shaped perfusion deficits which are rarely symmetrical in size, intensity of uptake and localization. Basal ganglia perfusion deficits may often be identified. Quantification of size and amplitude of perfusion deficits correlates with severity of disease. Larger and more pronounced deficits are found in more severe cases. Quantification alone does not separate DAT from MID. This is inferred by the pattern of distribution of the abnormalities.

# Cerebrovascular disease – stroke

*Example A9*

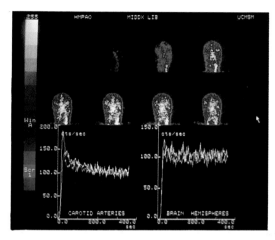

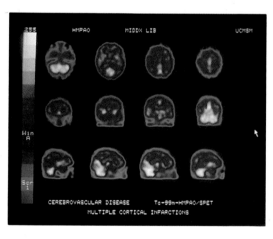

*Description* – This is a study from a 52-year-old male with cerebrovascular disease and known severe right common carotid artery stenosis. The top part shows the initial angiographic distribution of tracer through the carotid arteries and cerebral circulation with time-activity curves displayed from regions of interest in the carotids and cerebral hemispheres. This forms the basis for the calculation of CBF using some mathematical algorithms and brain perfusion indices. In this particular case there is very poor visualization of the right carotid artery, whilst there is no significant decrease or delay on the time-activity curve for the right hemisphere. The circle of Willis is patent. However multiple small wedge-shaped perfusion deficits are seen in the right hemisphere (frontal and parietal) with SPET, shown in the lower part.

*Comments*

* Using a large field-of-view gamma camera and initial angiographic distribution of the brain perfusion tracer via the aortic arch and carotid circulations it is possible to obtain quantitative data on CBF. This is of paramount importance in follow-up studies and may demonstrate some value in the prognosis of cerebro-vascular disease if regional rCBF values can be calculated for the infarct and penumbra areas.

  At present, structural imaging (CT or MRI) is imperative in acute stroke to rule out haemorrhagic infarction. SPET is of some value to study follow-up, therapeutic effects and possibly to establish prognosis when early studies (less than 6 h post onset) are carried out.

# Cerebrovascular disease – stroke

*Example A10*

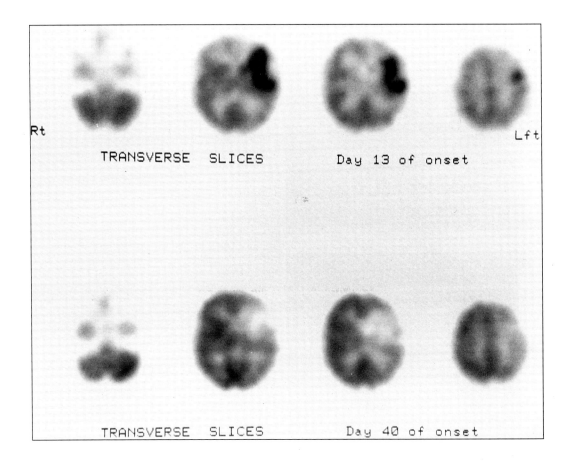

*Description* – This B&W figure shows two brain perfusion SPET studies (only horizontal slices) from a 43-year-old female with cerebrovascular disease and an infarction in the territory of distribution of the left middle cerebral artery. The upper row illustrates the so-called 'reactive hyperaemia' in the watershed areas between the territories of distribution of the middle, anterior and posterior cerebral arteries, seen by day 13 post onset of the cerebral vascular insult, most probably embolic (CT was normal at day 1 of onset). By day 40 post onset there is a large and single perfusion deficit in the territory of the middle cerebral artery, involving mainly the dorsolateral frontal cortex and less intensely the parietal cortex.

*Comments*
• Late hyperaemia, particularly in the watershed areas, has been taken as a sign of poor prognosis.

# Epilepsy (interictal)

## *Example A11*

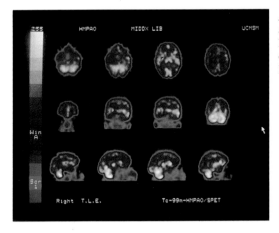

*Description* – This brain perfusion SPET study from a 26-year-old female with right temporal lobe epilepsy shows a single abnormality seen as a decrease of the regional brain perfusion to the right temporal lobe during the interictal period.

## *Example A12*

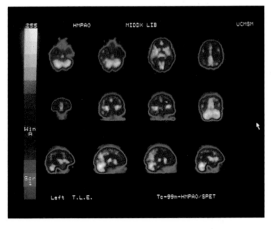

*Description* – This brain perfusion SPET study from a 35-year-old male with left temporal lobe epilepsy shows a single abnormality seen as a decrease of the regional brain perfusion to the left temporal lobe during the interictal period.

*Comments*

- In the interictal period of focal epilepsy, SPET studies demonstrate areas of decreased perfusion rates that may be uni- or multifocal. The sensitivity of interictal brain perfusion SPET in the detection of the epileptic focus has been reported to be relatively low.

# Epilepsy (ictal)

*Example A13*

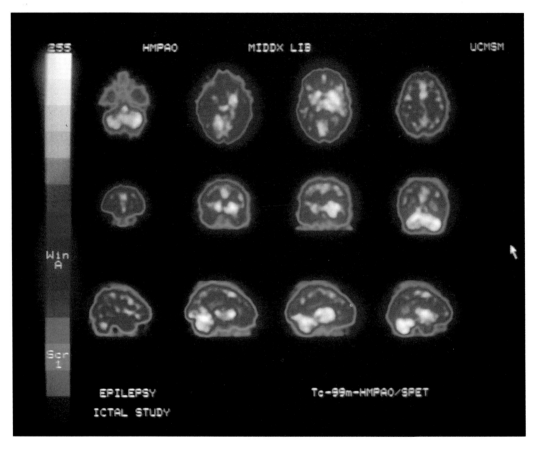

*Description* – This brain perfusion SPET study from a 28-year-old male shows a small area of increased tracer concentration corresponding to increased regional brain perfusion in the transition between the inferior frontal and superior and anterior temporal cortex on the left hemisphere during an ictal period. In addition, areas of reduced regional brain perfusion are seen in the right temporal lobe.

*Comments*

- Ictal SPET studies are more sensitive for detecting foci of epilepsy than interictal studies. The combination of interictal and ictal brain perfusion SPET studies appears to be able to detect more than 95% of the epileptic foci confirmed surgically.

  Studies with larger series of patients and with post-surgery follow-up are warranted in order to establish the role of brain perfusion SPET studies in the pre-surgical evaluation of patients with focal epilepsy.

# Epilepsy (temporal lobe reorientation)

*Example A14*

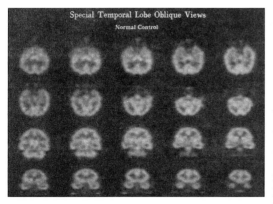

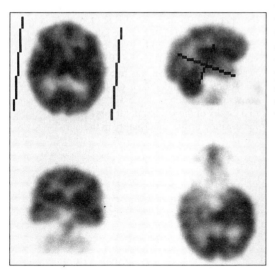

*Description* – This B&W figure demonstrates the steps followed by the reorientation process to achieve better visualization of the temporal lobes. From the initial axial reconstruction of one-pixel slices, the sagittal plane is drawn by joining the anterior with the posterior interhemispheric grooves. On a parasagittal plane through one of the temporal lobes a line is drawn parallel to the inferior temporal cortex to obtain the long axis of the temporal lobe. This gives origin to horizontal temporal lobe slices (bottom right) which open the temporal cortex and create a clear distinction between the medial and lateral cortices, as well as the anterior tip of the temporal lobe. A line perpendicular to the previous one enables the display of modified coronal slices for a better identification of the medial, lateral and inferior cortices of the temporal lobes (bottom left).

*Comments*

• To improve the detection of foci of epilepsy it is important to maximize our reporting performance. Quality assurance (instrumentation, radiotracer and protocols) has to be first on the list of priorities. However, technical details, like the one described for the reorientation of the temporal lobe, may play an important role.

# Herpes virus encephalitis

*Example A15*

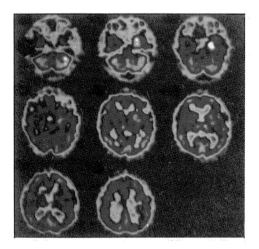

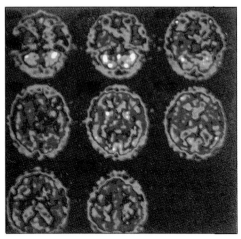

*Description* – This plate shows two brain perfusion SPET studies (horizontal slices only) from a 63-year-old man with herpes virus encephalitis. The first (top) was carried out 6 days post onset of the disease (mainly temperature and seizure) and demonstrates the characteristic increase of the radiotracer deposition in the medial cortex of the left temporal lobe, as if it were an ictal study from a patient with focal epilepsy. However, when the SPET investigation was performed, this patient was free of seizures. The second study was undertaken 60 days post onset and shows decreased regional brain perfusion to the medial cortex of the left temporal lobe, exactly the same localization as the abnormality in the initial study.

*Comments*
- The findings of focal increase of the tracer accumulation in the medial cortex of one of the temporal lobes in a patient with fever and presumptive diagnosis of herpes virus encephalitis (HVE) significantly increases the probability of HVE final diagnosis.

# Tumour

*Example A16*

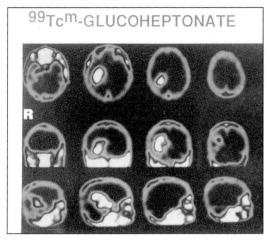

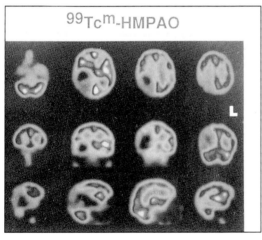

*Description* – This figure shows two SPET studies from a 47-year-old female with an intracerebral glioblastoma. The study on the top is a conventional blood–brain barrier SPET study depicting the disrupted blood–brain barrier in the right temporo-parietal lobes (increased tracer accumulation). The study on the bottom demonstrates no deposition of the brain perfusion tracer in the tumour. The area of reduced regional brain perfusion to the temporo-parietal area appears larger in the brain perfusion than the blood–brain barrier SPET because of the presence of peritumoural oedema.

*Comments*
- The majority of tumours demonstrate low brain perfusion tracer deposition due to disruption of the blood–brain barrier. However some reports have shown a wide variability of tumour concentration, from lower to higher than normal grey matter. No relationship has been established between either grade of tumour or vascularity to degree of tumour uptake.

# Tumour

## *Example A17*

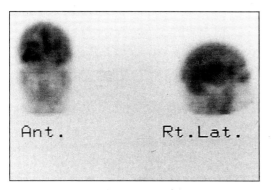

*Description* – This is a brain perfusion SPET study of a 28-year-old female with an arteriovenous malformation (AVM) of the right temporal lobe. Despite the intense vascularity of this abnormality the final uptake and retention of brain perfusion tracers is significantly reduced because there is no brain tissue. The tracer arriving from the arterial supply is directed into the venous system and systemic circulation without uptake and retention in the tumour. The coronal slices clearly demonstrate the tumour in the body of the right temporal lobe with shift of the surrounding structures (mass effect).

## *Example A18*

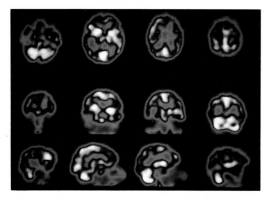

*Description* – These two planar images show a well-circumscribed area of increase of the brain perfusion tracer uptake and retention in a neuroblastoma of the right orbit.

*Comments*

• Although highly vascular, AVMs demonstrate no tracer retention due to the lack of blood–brain barrier integrity. The abundance of neuronal and/or glial cells in neural crest tumours gives rise to the uptake and retention of brain perfusion tracers similarly to the central nervous system.

Unfortunately there have been no reports of the possible utility of brain perfusion tracers for the post-therapy follow-up of patients with tumours of the neural crest.

# Neuroreceptors (D₂ dopamine)

*Example A19*

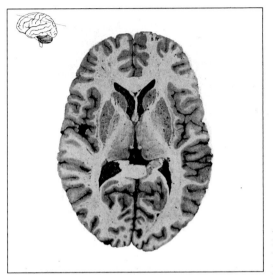

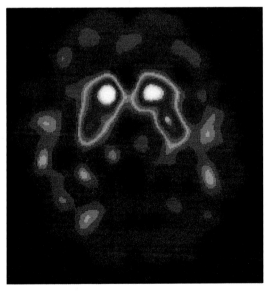

*Description* – Radioligands for the D$_2$ dopamine neuroreceptor accumulate in the striatum, the head of the caudate nucleus and putamen on both hemispheres. In this figure an anatomical drawing is shown for comparison with a single horizontal slice through the basal ganglia to highlight the uptake of a D$_2$ dopamine neuroreceptor ligand in the caudate nuclei and putamen.

*Comment*

- The specific binding to the striatal structures characteristically marks the availability of the D$_2$ dopamine neuroreceptors.

# Neuroreceptor (D₂ dopamine)

*Example A20*

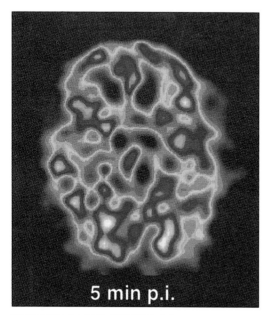

5 min p.i.

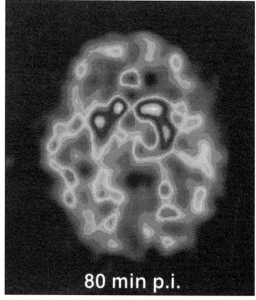

80 min p.i.

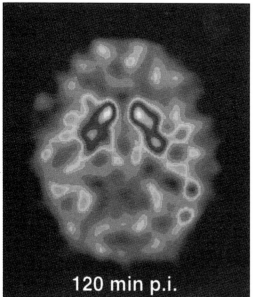

120 min p.i.

*Description* – This figure illustrates the temporal sequential change in the distribution of the D₂ dopamine neuroreceptor ligand in a normal volunteer (28-year-old female) from 5 min to 2 h post injection. Only three horizontal slices at the level of the basal ganglia and parallel to the AC–PC line are shown. The first slice (5 min post injection) displays the initial perfusion-like image with non-specific distribution of the radioligand. The second and third slices (80 min and 2 h post injection respectively) demonstrate the specific bindings of the D₂ dopamine neuroreceptor marker to the striatum (caudate nuclei and putamen).

*Comments*

• If one can demonstrate that the initial images (5–10 min post injection) are truly representative of regional brain perfusion, a more sensitive method of calculating the specific binding may be obtainable. It takes time for the specific binding to be selectively identified (usually between 1 and 2 h post injection).

# Neuroreceptors (D2 dopamine)

*Example A21*

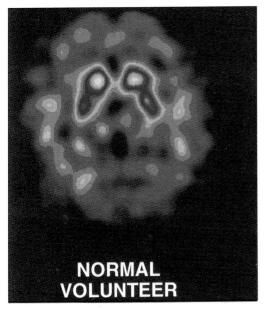

*Description* – This figure shows a comparison between the striatum specific binding of $D_2$ dopamine neuroreceptor radioligand in a schizophrenic patient and an age-matched normal volunteer. Poor patient co-operation significantly interferes with the SPET study quality. However, there is a significant difference observed between the naive and antipsychotic studies of the schizophrenic patient. Under antipsychotic therapy the specific binding of the $D_2$ dopamine neuroreceptor ligand is drastically reduced, demonstrating receptor non-availability.

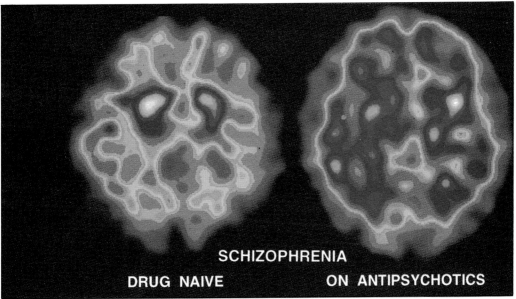

*Comments*

- There is potential for a better *in vivo* titration of the antipsychotic therapy than the one obtained from plasmatic or serum levels of antipsychotic drugs.

# Neuroreceptors (benzodiazepine)

*Example A22*

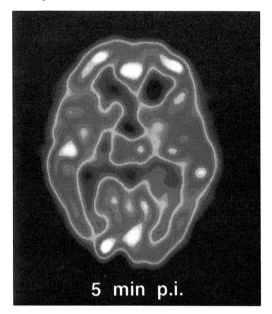

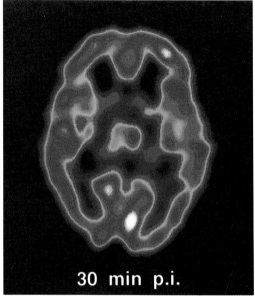

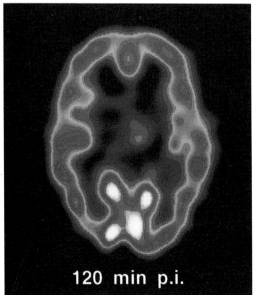

*Description* – This figure demonstrates the time-sequence changes observed during a SPET study of the distribution of the benzodiazepine receptor neuroligand on a 64-year-old normal male. The initial image (5 min post injection) shows a perfusion-like pattern, whilst the other two demonstrate the progressive clearance from the non-specific binding structures (striatum) and retention in the specific binding cortical grey matter (30 min and particularly 2 h post injection).

*Comments*

- Some studies have emphasized the possible role of iomazenil interictal SPECT in the localization of epileptic foci.
  However, its true clinical potential needs further investigation.

# Multiple tracer studies

*Example A23*

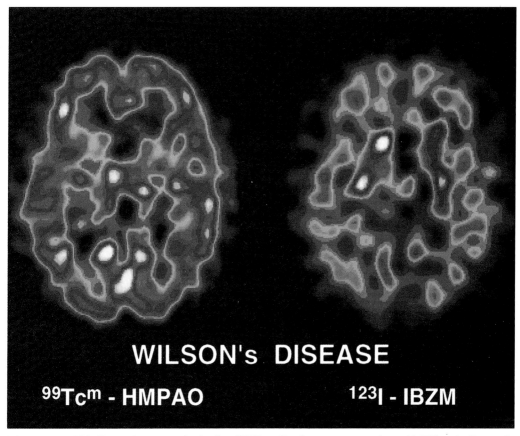

**WILSON's DISEASE**

**99Tcm - HMPAO**          **123I - IBZM**

*Description* – This figure shows two single slice SPET studies from a young patient with Wilson's disease. In this condition abnormal amounts of copper are deposited in the striatum giving rise to a disabling movement disorder of difficult management.

The image on the left hand side is from a brain perfusion study (single slice at the level of the basal ganglia) and shows marked reduction of the regional perfusion values to the striatum, particularly the caudate nuclei. The image on the right hand side is from a $D_2$ dopamine neuroreceptor study (similar level to the perfusion study), and shows marked reduction of the specific binding of the radioligand.

*Comments*

- In neurological conditions affecting the striatum (e.g. cortico-basal degeneration, Huntington's and Wilson's disease), it is essential to study brain perfusion and dopamine neuroceptor availability, due to the primary abnormality in the striatal neurons, and the possible consequent cortical deafferentiation, frequently observed.

These studies may be important to differentiate traits from state of the disease and possibly to assess therapeutic follow-up.

# Subject Index